THE
JOY
CHOICE

HOW TO FINALLY ACHIEVE
LASTING CHANGES IN EATING AND EXERCISE

MICHELLE SEGAR, PhD

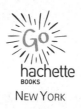

hachette
BOOKS

NEW YORK

Copyright © 2022 by Michelle Segar

Cover design by Terri Sirma
Interior art copyright © Michelle Segar; Design by Chris Bidlack/Bidlack Creative Group
Cover copyright © 2022 by Hachette Book Group, Inc.

Hachette Go, an imprint of Hachette Books
Hachette Book Group
1290 Avenue of the Americas
New York, NY 10104
HachetteGo.com
Facebook.com/HachetteGo
Instagram.com/HachetteGo

First Paperback Edition: July 2023

Hachette Books is a division of Hachette Book Group, Inc.

The Hachette Go and Hachette Books name and logos are trademarks of Hachette Book Group, Inc.

The publisher is not responsible for websites (or their content) that are not owned by the publisher.

Library of Congress Control Number: 2021952285

ISBNs: 978-0-306-82607-8 (hardcover); 978-0-306-82608-5 (paperback); 978-0-306-82609-2 (ebook)

Printed in the United States of America

LSC-C

Printing 1, 2023

For everyone who has struggled to adopt healthy eating and regular physical activity in ways that are sustainable and nurturing. I wrote this book to help you understand why it's not your fault and guide you to new science and simple tools that can help you turn this around in feel-good, self-affirming, and lasting ways.

CONTENTS

INTRODUCTION
IT'S NOT YOUR FAULT

DOES THIS SEQUENCE OF EVENTS SEEM AT ALL FAMILIAR?

YOU CREATE YOUR IDEAL PLAN IN
A MOTIVATION BUBBLE

BUT THEN LIFE HAPPENS!

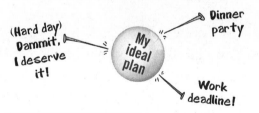

LIFE BURSTS THE MOTIVATION BUBBLE

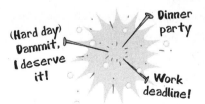

If so, you're not alone and you're in good company.

We typically initiate a change in eating or exercise or other self-care behaviors in what I call a "motivation bubble." It might be New Year's resolutions time, an upcoming wedding, or some image we see on social media that inspires us to start an ambitious eating or exercise project, again. We are filled with inspiration, commitment, determination, and energy. At *these* moments, our goals feel very attainable and we have a sincere belief that *this time we will really do it!* But at this point, our motivation bubble feels like it's in a completely different orbit from the other parts of our busy lives; as soon as this giant (yet fragile) motivation bubble comes into contact with *any* everyday conflict or challenge, it easily bursts. And when it does, our intended eating and exercise plans go right down the drain. This happens again, and again, and again.

When my clients start working with me, they tell me that it's their fault they can never stick with their healthy eating and exercise plans and goals. Beyond self-blame, they lament their lack of will-power and assert that *if they just had more* self-control, they'd achieve lasting success.

They couldn't be more wrong.

It's not their fault, just like it's not yours. We've been told a sin-gular story of behavior change that sets most of us up to start and stop, and start and stop, but never to sustain. This story is simplistic and misguides us to focus on the wrong things, like needing more self-control. Or it seduces us into believing that the latest exercise fad, popular diet, or trending behavior-change strategy is our golden ticket to *finally* getting it right. Yet, as you likely know, while these things work for some, they don't work for the majority of us. Let's talk about why.

Whatever the reason, season, or event that motivates us to start anew and may even help us succeed for a while, sooner or later life just happens! Work gets busy, an aging parent needs extra care, our kids and animals have unanticipated needs…Our hoped for, well-intended eating choices or exercise plans will eventually face a conflict. And *this conflict* often turns out to be the culprit, the mundane thing that derails our grand plan, kicking us right off the path of lasting change.

The behavior change story most of us have learned *hasn't focused on* these conflicts that never stop arising, nor has it taught us how to avoid or overcome them. I call these conflicts "choice points," and they are the real place of power for achieving lasting changes in eating and exercise.

If lasting change is what you're after, I'm here to help.

If you could find a simple and fun approach for overcoming these in-the-moment conflicts that derail our best intentions would you be interested in learning more about it? Welcome to *The Joy Choice*!

But first, I'm going to say something that may genuinely shock you.

A WHOLE NEW WORLD

Now.

If you're like most of my clients, weight loss probably figures into your behavior change goals in some way. One of the biggest things I've learned about creating lasting changes in eating and exercise behavior is that hitching them to a weight-loss goal can't be sustained by most people. I know this may sound counter to everything we've been taught, but research suggests that if you want to stick with your desired changes in eating and exercise, it will be unlikely if weight loss is your primary goal. But don't worry—*The Joy Choice* is here to help you navigate this new territory.

In *The Joy Choice*, you'll discover the science-based and real-world reasons that weight-loss goals inadvertently *thwart desired changes in eating and exercise* for so many of us. You'll also learn how to move from this roller coaster of failure into the cycle of sustainable success. But make no mistake. This book is not about changing our behavior. It's about what we can do to achieve *lasting* change.

And that starts with ditching what decades of personal experience shows leads to false hopes and eventual self-sabotage and replacing it with what the emerging science and my work with clients suggests is powerful enough to change the way we think and feel and drive the consistent choices that favor healthy eating and regular exercise. *The Joy Choice* rewrites the story of behavior change with this new and delightfully counterintuitive science showing that play, positive experiences, and affirming who we are at our core are the actual ingredients of achieving lasting change.

Rule-based, perfection-seeking, weight-focused behavior-change approaches do get us started and inflate our motivation bubble. But they don't stand a *lasting* chance in the crazy-busy context of our other daily priorities and needs. Many of us bounce like billiard balls between career responsibilities, schoolwork, household tasks, medical appointments, aging parents, our own parenting responsibilities, and the list goes on. The resulting stress, fatigue, anxiety, and overwhelming quantity of daily tasks and decisions create cognitive overload (too many things to do!) and decision fatigue (too many choices to make!).

As I thought about the idea that the stress of daily life could mimic the attention-scattering thinking caused by conditions like ADHD (attention deficit/hyperactivity disorder), I realized that the issues that some of my clients—and maybe you, too—grapple with *reflect challenges we all face under stress*: getting distracted by unexpected demands, feeling overwhelmed by options, making the impulsive choice rather than the one we had planned, and ultimately giving up in despair of ever reaching our goals, *again*. Can you relate?

The story of behavior change we've been told all these years is not really the best way to behavioral sustainability. Well, then, what is?

THE PERFECT *IMPERFECT* SOLUTION

Behavioral sustainability is the result we want, but to do that, we need to know how to make the consistent decisions that underlie that lofty objective. When we start a change, we tend to focus on the future goal that it is in service of achieving. But change does not happen in the future. Change happens in *each moment*, with the choices and compromises we make when faced with the challenges of daily life: An urgent call cut into your planned exercise class! Should you work out for a shorter time than you'd planned? Replace the class with five minutes of dancing with your kids? Drop the whole idea of exercise today? We can't stop these unexpected conflicts from arising, but we can learn how to stop them from derailing our greater goals!

This is the place our attention needs to be: on the front lines of the conflict between our well-crafted eating or exercise plan and the messy, frequent real-life circumstances that challenge it. In *The Joy Choice*, you'll hear stories from my work with clients and industry that will show you how to use simple strategies for making the choices that take us easily and joyfully *through* the dizzying swirl of conflict-induced distraction, which used to derail us, to the other side: sustaining our healthy eating and exercise goals *within the context of our full set of daily priorities and needs.*

This is the choice that keeps you on the path of lasting change, and this is the premise, and the promise, of *The Joy Choice.*

THE JOY CHOICE: THE STORY YOU'VE BEEN WAITING FOR

The Joy Choice transforms the high-stakes hard work of "sticking with the program" into something new: a fresh and joyful approach for navigating the daily decisions and conflicts we face about what to eat or how to fit our exercise in and still meet work, family, and other life needs. And this profound change changes everything. *The Joy Choice* celebrates and supports our brain's innate self-management system for making the consistent healthy eating and exercise decisions that underlie achieving lasting change. By turning the behavior change story on its head, we get straight to the heart of lasting change.

The first chapters of *The Joy Choice* reveal the hidden barriers to lasting change we so often encounter, and how we can understand and avoid them. You'll learn:

+ the surprising reasons that habits created for eating and exercise so often crash when they come up against real life;
+ the disruptive effects that our crazy-busy lives have on our brain's ability to manage our choices, plans, and goals; and
+ the ins and outs of our four primary *decision disruptors*, the hidden traps like temptation and rebellion that we fall into time and time again.

In the second part of the book, we'll move directly into the comprehensive and joyful solution: *The Joy Choice* graphic-based strategies and decision shortcuts that let us escape those past traps and make the choices that keep us moving forward, finally achieving lasting change. You'll learn:

+ three science-based decision-support strategies—Simplify, Play, and Choose Joy—that will help us quiet the mental noise and clear the decks for effective decision making through joy, ease, and flexbility;
+ to use the fun and easy three-step POP! decision tool that enables us to effortlessly navigate the in-the-moment conflicts our eating and exercise plans face by helping us focus, open up to new options, and pick the Joy Choice, the meaningful com-

promise that *keeps us on track* so we can stay in sync with ourselves and the people and things that matter most; and

* the simple, tactical thinking that underlies lasting change.

IN THE JOY CHOICE, I'M PROPOSING THAT WE SHIFT OUR GAZE
from the far North Star of idealized aspirations, stop blaming
ourselves, and chart our own unique journey through *right now*—
exploring with curiosity, humor, and compassion the messy, noisy,
and predictably unpredictable life that belongs to each and every one
of us. We will quiet the noise and confusion and put our attention
where it really matters: in the moment of choice, armed with the
new thinking and practical strategies we need to master this moment
with purpose, play, and joy.

As you read *The Joy Choice*, you will learn how to retake the reins
of your own choices and goals and discover your new story of lasting
behavior change—this time, with a happy ending.

The Joy Choice is yours.

one

IS THE POWER OF HABITS ALL IT'S CRACKED UP TO BE FOR HEALTHY EATING AND EXERCISE?

A FEW YEARS AGO, I BEGAN TO NOTICE THAT MORE AND MORE OF MY CLIents were asking me to help them develop a "new habit" for sticking with a diet or healthy eating plan or making exercise a permanent part of their daily life. "I don't know what's wrong," they say. "I know it should be easy, but something always seems to get in the way and I get sidetracked. Can you help figure this out?"

Well, yes and no. Let me explain.

ARE YOU A HABITER OR AN UNHABITER?

Tuesday, five a.m., the middle of winter, and our hundred-year-old house in Ann Arbor, Michigan, is dark and cold. I am huddled under the covers when my husband's alarm rings, as it does every morning. Jeff quickly turns it off, climbs out of bed, and heads for the basement, already dressed in workout clothes so he doesn't have to think about anything other than starting his exercise. For decades, he has biked for forty-five minutes, lifted weights, showered, eaten breakfast, and headed off to work, refreshed and ready for his day. He is a true believer in the power of his habit, and for good reason: it works for him. Can you relate to this?

Let me be the first to say that I cannot. And perhaps you can't either.

You probably know someone like Jeff, for whom this type of habit actually works. But I'm going to come right out and say it: If you are hoping to easily incorporate behaviors like daily exercise, more thoughtful eating, or other self-care behaviors like meditation into your busy, noisy, wonderful, frustrating, and complicated daily life, forming lifelong habits is probably not going to work for you.

Wait—what?

Some people are innately more wired for disciplined living, while others struggle to harness their focus and self-control. Before you embark on a new lifestyle change that you intend to sustain, it's important to recognize whether you are more like what I call a *habiter*, like Jeff, or an *unhabiter*, like me.

Take a moment to look over the following statements, and check off the ones you agree with:

❑ I am very disciplined and organized.

❑ I stick to my plan even when I am tempted; I do not make impulsive choices.

❑ My days run according to schedule, with rare exceptions.

❑ I don't have any inner conflicts or ambivalence about eating healthy foods or exercising—I am 100 percent on board.

☐ I tend to rely on someone else to manage many of my daily needs (e.g., schedule meetings, transport children, make meals, organize social events, etc.).

How did you do?

These statements reflect qualities and circumstances that enable habits to form—a disciplined personality, low internal conflict, and stable daily structures with low levels of unanticipated needs. If you agreed with most or all of the boxes on this list, you're probably a habiter: It's much more likely you'll be able to form and stick with habits as a behavioral strategy for achieving and sustaining your health, fitness, and self-care goals.

If you found yourself unable to agree with these statements, or disagreed with most of them, forming lifelong habits for changes in eating and exercise is less likely to work for you. You're an unhabiter, and this book is for you.

ARE HABITS REALLY THE BEST SOLUTION FOR LASTING CHANGES IN EATING AND EXERCISE?

Jeff and I have a lot in common, and some basic differences. Like me, he's a scientist. Like me, he loves to eat great food, play Ping-Pong with our son, and hang out with friends and family. Unlike me, he's a naturally disciplined, well-organized person who keeps everything neat and clean, plans his upcoming work-related needs every Sunday, and always manages to do what needs to be done, even if it means skimping on sleep.

As a person who values rest and is comfortable with leaving a few dishes in the sink, I find Jeff's ease with sticking with complex habits like exercise and surviving on less sleep both frustrating and enviable. The idea of incorporating this seeming effortlessness into my own routine is very attractive, and I have been successful with making habits of some simple tasks (notably, flossing at night, checking our dog's water bowl in the morning, and drinking a glass of water myself as soon as I wake up). Habits do serve an important role in our lives, and they help us achieve certain things without effort or thought, enabling us to save our conscious thinking for the times we need it most.[1] But I am also aware that this does not mean habits are the answer for sticking with the more complex behaviors and goals that so often end up in our New Year's resolutions.

The very process that makes habits so valuable for simple, mechanical behaviors like making coffee in the morning or taking your meds at the same time and place every day also makes them unworkable for many people who want to adopt more complex lifestyle behaviors—like getting to the gym regularly, or avoiding junk food— that they can sustain within the challenges of daily life. To really understand why habiters and unhabiters might benefit from different behavior change solutions, it's important to understand what habits really are.

WHAT ARE HABITS, ANYWAY?

When I ask people how they define a habit, the most common response is "doing something with regularity." Does that mean every day? Most of the time? This is a pretty vague description for a habit. To actually create an automatic habit, it's important to determine precisely what you want to do and when you want to do it, such as put your keys on a hook by the door as soon as you enter your home from work.

You might recognize this idea because popular books generally teach us to form habits based on this more formal and precise definition of a habit: *performing an action reflexively, without the need to think or exert self-control*—theoretically saving time, saving willpower, and saving our brain power for other tasks.[2] What these books have been advocating for is specifically referred to as *habit formation*. But for habit formation to work, it needs to meet a very important requirement: *it has to occur within a stable context*.[3] Habit formation is the topic of a lot of research, fuels current debate, and is also used to design many healthy behavior apps, so it's worth taking a moment to understand.

Habit formation is often described as a three-part process:

- The *cue* is the trigger or cause of the habit (e.g., Jeff's wake-up alarm).
- The *behavior* is the actual action—the desired habit (e.g., riding the bike).
- The *reward* is some type of positive experience or feeling associated with the behavior (e.g., feeling accomplished, refreshed).

Together, these three elements constitute a *habit loop* (as shown in the figure), which is necessary to form a habit that sticks.[4]

THE HABIT LOOP

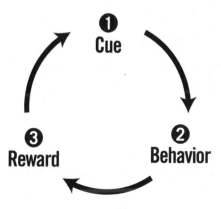

❶ Cue

❷ Behavior

❸ Reward

Habit formation of this type requires one very important condition: it needs to occur in a *stable*, unchanging context. This requirement is so central to the ultimate success of forming habits that Wendy Woods, a leading researcher of habits, says, "Variety weakens habit...variety is the enemy of stable contexts...If you are not arranging your life to reliably, unfailing, cue your habit, then that habit will never take hold."[5] Unfortunately, when it comes to eating and exercise, the real world rarely plays along with this scenario.

The popular habit approach derives from pioneering psychologist William James (1842–1910). He wrote a book called *Habit* that promoted the value of automating our days through habits so as to free our minds for our most important work.[6] This advice came long before our lives were continually interrupted by email, texting, social media, online dating, not to mention parents who have to juggle managing their children's screens, gaming, and social media, drive kids to numerous classes, games, and parties, and make time to watch the latest streaming must-see series. Even within this context, habits work well for many simple tasks and for people like Jeff, who are naturals.

But the currently popular narrative advocates habit formation as a solution that can work for anybody and any behavior, and it has become a popular part of the behavior change story. There are some interesting science-based reasons that forming habits for eating and exercise works for habiters, but is not likely to work for me and others who are unhabiters.

EXAMINING FOUR COMMON ASSUMPTIONS ABOUT HABITS FOR HEALTHY EATING AND EXERCISE

My clients sometimes come to me saying that they did something wrong because they can't make habits work for their lifestyle goals, continuing the self-blame game. They believe that they *should be able to* form an exercise or healthy eating "habit" because they hear everyone talking about it, their family and friends and online influencers. But these beliefs are based on four common assumptions about "everybody" that don't hold up under scrutiny.

Assumption 1. Everyone can form habits.

Popular thinking holds that habits can work for everyone. But there are several reasons that this thinking doesn't hold up when it comes to forming habits for complex lifestyle behaviors.

First, you may be surprised to discover that much of the research on human habits has not been conducted on a typical sample of "everyone." Instead, these studies often use limited (*not* representative) populations, including specific groups that might be more inclined toward habit formation, like active members in a fitness club or college students who may have less on their daily plates.

So, what's wrong with using college students in studies about forming lasting lifestyle habits? Consider this: The vast majority of university students at four-year institutions are between the ages of eighteen and twenty-four, are mostly single,[7] so their lives are likely to have fewer responsibilities and be less logistically complicated than those of working adults. In fact, a highly cited academic study on how long it takes people to develop habit *"automaticity,"* performing an action on autopilot without the need to think about doing it, was conducted mostly among postgraduate students (average age twenty-seven) in the United Kingdom.[8]

The ninety-six students who enrolled were asked to choose one new behavior to perform daily in the same context (e.g., after dinner) for twelve weeks. They chose to form new healthy habits related to either drinking water, eating, meditation, or exercise. This study found that it took sixty-six days, on average, for habit automaticity to form.

Research helps advance our knowledge. And this interesting study is no exception by contributing to what we know about habits and automaticity. This research, and its sixty-six-day finding, are heavily cited across academia and industry. Yet there are some reasons to be cautious about generalizing these findings beyond this study. The biggest issue relates to the wide variability in time participants took to achieve automaticity, ranging from 18 to 254 days. This range, and the 66-day average derived from it, is so large that it is hard to justify as a rule of thumb to use outside of this study. Also, about half of the graduate students in this study didn't do their target behavior enough to achieve the automaticity status that the study was about. In their conclusion, the authors noted that "even in this study where the participants were motivated to create habits, approximately half did not perform the behavior consistently enough to achieve habit status." Even though the authors clearly acknowledged their study limitations, the sixty-six-day habit formation stat is often promoted as an established fact. As with so many other behavior-change targets, when we aim for what we've been told and it doesn't hold, we are left feeling like a failure, again.

When we are trying to understand how to form habits, or other techniques aiming to create sustainable lifestyle changes, we need to be careful about generalizing research conducted among university students to the general population of adults. Although some students have jobs and families, they may also have fewer complex responsibilities related to caring for and managing family- and work-related needs.

Second, research suggests that certain personalities succeed better than others at forming habits. Not surprisingly, people who tend to be innately disciplined and have high self-control (like my husband) are better at forming habits that those of us who don't share those traits.[9] When I speak about this in presentations, most people jump to the conclusion that the only reason some people have trouble forming new exercise and healthy eating habits is that they don't have the innate self-disciplined personality. But, as you'll soon learn, this is not true.

Assumption 2. Our internal conflicts about eating and exercise do not affect our ability to form automatic habits for eating and exercise.

One reason the idea of habit formation is so attractive is that the mechanistic idea of automatic behavior sidesteps the guilt, shame, resistance, rebellion, and other internal conflicts that so often pull the plug on our eating and exercise resolutions. It's easy to assume that once it's installed—out of sight and out of mind—the habit will easily override any complicated feelings about exercise or healthy eating we may have. But there are some compelling reasons as to why this is a false assumption.

Whether we realize it or not, we often change our behavior to conform to cultural pressures (to get "our younger body back" or to please our partners or parents) or on doctor's orders (to drop pounds or exercise more and eat better to improve our health). Yet, when we try to make these "sensible" changes, many of us encounter a feeling of internal pressure and obligation. These forces are often unconscious but they still exert pressure, so it's no wonder that conflict kicks in. This inner conflict exerts itself in many ways: Long-standing shame about our bodies bubbles up to sabotage our good intentions, leading us to avoid the punishing, high-intensity exercise we think we *must* do to burn calories. Resentment over the (often self-imposed) restrictions we now have to follow *actually motivates us to rebel against them,* and we might even find ourselves choosing to eat a box of cookies without realizing we had taken it out of the drawer, dammit! We may even cancel our annual physical so we don't have to hear our doctor's (well-meaning) warning to lose weight or risk getting diabetes.

Let's be real: How many people *don't* experience inner conflicts with making changes in eating and exercise? We may feel that our motives are solely our own, our goals are simple, and habit formation is what will get us there quickly. But the fact is, many, if not most of us, have a great deal of psychological conflict wrapped up with dietary change and exercise, and habits can't make this conflict disappear.

Importantly, there are theories about, and research showing, that these types of inner conflicts will almost inevitably spoil our best intentions. *Self-determination theory*[10] proposes that if we do not feel aligned with our goals or choices (for example, joining a gym because it's the *en vogue* place to work out, but we hate going because it makes us feel bad about ourselves), this not only demotivates us but can pile on guilt and shame. *Reactance theory*[11] would contend that when we feel pressured to exercise more or eat in healthier ways, especially from a "should," we are literally motivated to react against or do the *opposite of our intended action*—even *when we* are the ones who initiated the change.

Worse, these inner conflicts all too easily cause negative associations and ambivalence that inhibit our ability to experience the very positive rewards needed to drive the habit loop! These conflicts can lead to an internal friction, which disrupts the nonconscious automaticity that habits depend on to stick.[12] They also deplete us, leaving little energy to power through our ambivalence.[13]

Inner conflicts about trying to change our diet or exercise, whether conscious or not, put us at odds with our core self and lead us to sabotage rather than support sustainable behavior change. Believing that we should be able to "muscle through" our guilt and resentment just piles on more guilt, resentment, and conflict. Yet the common belief that we *should* be able to do this, and that habits will take us there, means that we rarely address these fundamental issues when we try to form a habit.

The bottom line? Habit formation demands a reliably stable context that makes our choices frictionless and depends on positive experiences. The turmoil created by inner conflict is anything but.

Assumption 3. It's possible to form an automatic habit for any lifestyle behavior.

This is the big one.

Here's how the thinking goes: Habits work so well for some behaviors that habit formation must be a great strategy for creating sustainable change for *any* behavior. It seems obvious that putting a health behavior on autopilot, as habit formation promises, will make the need for self-control obsolete—we make the healthy choice automatically, effortlessly, without a second thought. But this assumption is not correct.

It's true, we shouldn't *have* to think about simple behaviors like flossing daily or always putting the car keys in the same place. These are perfect for habit formation: the context is stable, the cue is the same, the reward is immediate, and repetition is built in. It's hard to imagine your key hook moving during the night and we floss inside the bathroom, a context known for few outside interruptions. The following graphic shows the relative ease of forming a flossing habit.

It's just you and your floss after (or before) brushing. No problem!

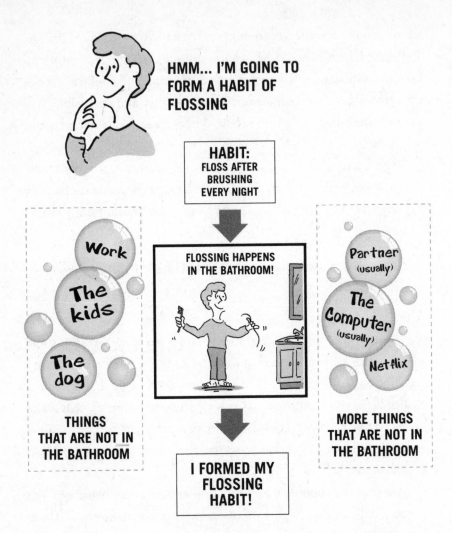

Now consider the many forces going *against* exercise habits: lack of desire, a rescheduled meeting, other people's needs, time to change clothes or shower...and these are only a few. Every day, even our best-laid exercise or eating plans get disrupted by life stuff (a family emergency, a bad day at work, low energy), or by the tug-of-war between our reflective self ("I should get to that spinning class.") and our reactive self ("I want to stream that show!").

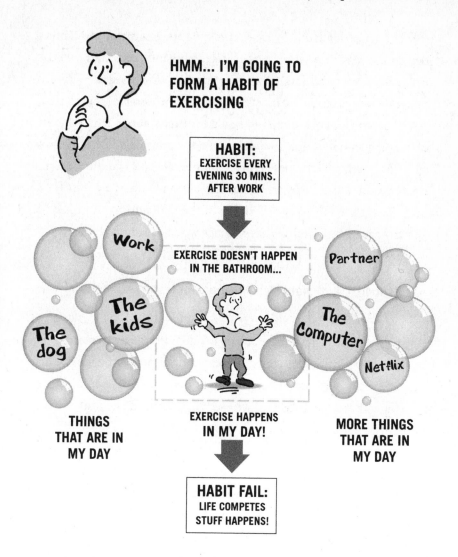

As this other graphic makes clear, in contrast to a simple behavior like flossing, our lifestyle behaviors are generally surrounded by the complexities inherent in the many contexts, people, and needs of our daily lives. Research suggests, for example, that even among people *with* strong exercise habits, a simple change in circumstances (like exercising in a different location) disrupts their exercise habit.[14]

The basis for habit formation comes from simple, mechanistic behaviors, so it's no surprise that disagreement exists over whether more complex behaviors (that is, behaviors with multiple subcomponents, like exercise) can even become automatic.[15] There's currently a healthy debate among habit scientists about the feasibility of automatic habits for complex lifestyle behaviors, including how they form, what is the best type of motivator, and whether internal circumstances can also cue them into action.[16] The jury is still out on this science, but we're still living in the real world and in need of healthy eating and exercise approaches we can count on.

Assumption 4. Automaticity is the ideal for lasting changes in healthy eating and exercise.

A much-touted virtue of habits is *automaticity*, or performing a behavior with little conscious awareness or effort.[17] The idea of acting reflexively, without any need for thought or work, sounds great, especially if you feel tired and stressed. Certainly, it's helpful in many parts of life, not least in helping us get out of bed and off to work in the morning.

We've known for a long time that we spend a lot of our day on autopilot and make many decisions unconsciously.[18] Some argue that because we *already* live so much of our lives this way, we might as well try to leverage this human tendency to form automatic habits for lifestyle behaviors like healthy eating and exercise too. Yet, given that automatic habits are vulnerable to disruption by deviation from the plan, those of us who have overlapping responsibilities (work, family, school, volunteering) and are also managing the logistics of numerous life arenas are unlikely to have the reliably stable life conditions required to form automatic habits for complex lifestyle behaviors.

Consider the almost daily schedule upheavals that require us to drop what we are doing or had planned to do and choose the best response *right now*, based on our actual circumstances in that moment. Autopilot can't help us here—we need conscious awareness to optimally solve the challenges we and our eating and exercise plans face.[19] In fact, the automatic and narrowed frame of mind cultivated in habit formation may actually *thwart* our real-world need to pivot, problem solve, and be sufficiently flexible to change course in the moment.[20]

Can the new "micro-habits" avoid the vulnerabilities of bigger ones? I'm a big fan of starting small, taking mini-steps, and staying realistic, as this new movement promotes.[21] If micro-habits refer to small steps, then that's different than the automatic habits being discussed here. But if we're talking about forming small *automatic* habits, their habit loop would be vulnerable to the same unexpected disruptions as their bigger counterparts.

In lives that present us with the continual need to improvise and negotiate, mounting science shows, paradoxically, that we need to be flexible (not rigid) if we hope to become consistent with exercise and healthy eating.[22] Eating and exercise habits are easily derailed by the unexpected: an urgent meeting at work that interferes with your gym plans, an abundance of "bad" food choices at your family get-together, a sudden snowstorm that makes your run impossible, your child's tummy ache the keeps you both in the house. These are far from unsolvable problems. Yet if we are relying on automatic responses when challenges arise to our hoped-for exercise and healthy eating habits, we may be unprepared and won't have the necessary consciousness in the moment to most effectively manage our competing obligations and make the best choice for our full set of needs—the task at hand, the people who rely on us, the time we have available—on the spot.

LIFE IS MESSY

So, here's the thing: Programming our eating and exercise choices to unfold effortlessly and without conscious thought sounds great in theory, but real life easily upsets the program. As a remedy, we could try streamlining our environments, getting rid of temptations, and arranging our lives—without any variation—to accommodate the automaticity needed for habit formation. These are great ideas, but this level of control over our lives is not always easy (or even possible) for many of us to achieve. In fact, there is little research support for the idea that habits can power *lasting* changes in lifestyle behaviors like eating or exercise.[23] What's more, studies aiming to corroborate this assumption have generally failed to do so, even among simple behaviors, such as flossing.[24]

Try as we might to smooth out the bumps in the road, life often seems to be nothing but one unexpected detour after the next. And like it or not, change is the enemy of reflexive, automatic habits. As we'll explore in the next chapter, research has found that these sorts of everyday changes and challenges can easily create a life context that overwhelms not only our ability to stick to the program we embarked on, but also our ability to make the in-the-moment choices that keep us on track with our goals.

two

CHANGING BEHAVIOR AMID THE CHAOS AND STRESS OF OUR CRAZY-BUSY LIVES

*C*HAOS IS FORMALLY DEFINED AS AN "UTTER STATE OF CONFUSION AND lack of order."[1] This may sound dramatic, but it reflects the reality in which many of us live. You may (or may not!) be surprised to learn just how relevant this is to behavior change.

Alison Miller, PhD, professor of health behavior and health education at the University of Michigan's School of Public Health, conducts research related to executive functioning, eating, and weight-related outcomes in family contexts. She sees chaos as impacting the behavior-change game in a couple of ways, especially when it comes to managing meal planning, prep, and implementation for a family. "If home life is generally chaotic and it's taking lots of attention and effort to manage the basics," she explains, "like getting up and out the door, it's hard to layer on 'extra' effort, like having ingredients for a healthy meal on hand—not to mention enough time and cognitive space to plan and prepare it. Furthermore, if the chaos is also causing stress, it may be more tempting to eat comfort foods as a strategy to regulate your emotions."[2] Even when we are committed, motivated, and striving toward a health or other type of self-care goal within a formal program, chaos and stress are such powerful forces that our best intentions and aspirations easily get blown away.

In fact, there is an actual measure used in research called the CHAOS Scale,[3] which assesses the level of *confusion*, *hubbub*, and *order* in the home as a key part of understanding exercise, eating, and health-related outcomes. The following are some of the questions from the twenty-two-item CHAOS measure. To get a snapshot of your own daily context, check off the statements that resonate with your own life:

☐ No matter how hard we try, we always seem to be running late.

☐ We almost always seem to be rushed.

☐ No matter what our family plans, it usually doesn't seem to work out.

☐ It's a real zoo in our home.

☐ It's so noisy, you can't hear yourself think in our home.

I don't know about you, but I can certainly relate! This not-unfamiliar level of noise and stress easily interferes with our concentration and our intentions. When we add a new resolve to eat differently or exercise more regularly, it's like throwing more logs on the fire. When life feels out of control, it's no surprise that we might grab for a new eating or exercise plan to restart our health project and get back to feeling good about ourselves. Yet it's also puzzling to think about how often we dive headfirst into a new lifestyle change without putting much thought into how it will fit within the *predictably* unpredictable reality of our complex daily lives and many roles.

Consider the relentless onslaught of unexpected daily interruptions and schedule changes, and how easy it is for these forces to thwart our best-laid plans. It can be this simple: You're dressed and headed out for your planned forty-minute bike ride when you get a calendar reminder that your report is due on the boss's desk on Monday. As you turn around and walk toward your computer your daughter walks in and says she's stressed about her math homework and needs your help *right now*. Then, your phone rings. You glance up at the clock and see that the time you allotted for your bike ride is already ticking away and you immediately feel defeated by the realization that you won't make it today—again.

LIVING IN AN ADHD WORLD

Now consider this: We live in a crazy-busy, unpredictable world that regularly upsets our brain's executive functioning, *the system that manages our complex, long-term goals.* The constant multitasking and pivoting of daily life easily overloads our thinking and disrupts our focus in ways that could be considered as mimicking the attention-scattering thinking that is caused by conditions like ADHD (attention deficit/hyperactivity disorder).[4]

Living with ADHD is accompanied by challenges related to all sorts of fundamental activities, such as prioritizing tasks, getting started on or finishing tasks, keeping track of belongings, forgetting what was just heard, and managing time, among other things.[5] Here's how one person with ADHD, writing in an online ADHD forum, describes daily life: "There are so many things that need

WAIT...
MY DAY LOOKS
MORE LIKE THIS:

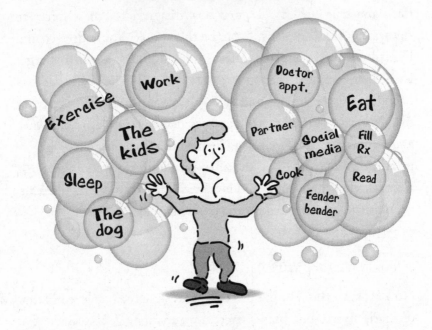

my attention every day. I feel like I'm always drowning in a maelstrom of stuff. It's hard to focus and achieve my goals with so many distractions!"

Sound familiar? I don't have ADHD like the person who spoke those words, and you might not either. Yet, like it or not, even those of us without ADHD can experience similar daily challenges. Our scattered focus becomes obvious when we try to add healthy behaviors into the mix. If we stand back and think about it objectively, why on earth would we even consider changing our lifestyles without giving serious consideration to the level of hubbub within which we hope our change will occur—and survive? Yet we do it over and over again, always wondering why we can't make it work.

As I've learned more about ADHD, especially the challenges related to successfully managing daily goals and needs and the feelings of being overwhelmed that make them worse, something fundamental dawned on me: *We don't need to have a condition like ADHD to have our brain-based self-management abilities worsened by living with chaos and complexity.*[6] Regardless of our own brain's baseline functioning, we know unequivocally that the human brain can't handle complexity very well because we have a finite amount of attention and other limited cognitive capacities. When you have many different bits of information, and you need to work with them, you have to simultaneously think about them as you make meaning with them. That's no small feat! Given how many things we have to manage combined with our brain's inherent limited bandwidth, we have little possibility of escaping detriments in our executive functioning that only get amplified by added stress and anxiety.

Make no mistake, I am not diagnosing everyone in the world with ADHD: For people with ADHD, things can seem extremely complex almost all the time. What I am saying is that extreme complexity and always being on the go challenges almost everyone.[7] With our inherent cognitive capacity limitations,[8] living with chaos and sudden, unexpected situations can't help but put our brain into a state where we are distracted, unfocused, unorganized, and impulsive—some of the core experiences that define what living with ADHD is like.

FALLING INTO THE GAP

This will probably not be news to you. The planner industry is booming, with a myriad of organizational techniques and specialized notebooks and apps to go along with them. Yet as much as we try to organize life with calendars and schedules, daily life presents unending challenges. We bounce between career responsibilities, schoolwork, household tasks, medical appointments, parenting, care for aging parents… The world outside our homes adds an unrelenting drumbeat of social media and news reports that sometimes seems impossible to escape. So, if you feel like your thoughts are scattered in a million directions and you wonder how you're going to fit in all your daily tasks—let alone how you're supposed to fit in a workout or eat the way you had planned—you're far from alone.

Researchers have looked at this very issue. A study published in the *Psychology of Sport and Exercise* investigated the effects of mental fatigue and overload on whether people decided to exercise.[9] Participants were randomized into one of two groups. One group completed a task that created a high cognitive demand, while the other group did a task that required less thinking. Afterward, mental fatigue was assessed. Then, participants were given the choice to exercise for twenty-two minutes or do a nonexercise task for twenty-two minutes. Results showed that participants in the high cognitive demand task reported increased mental fatigue, which in turn led them to perceive fewer benefits and higher costs to exercising, and ultimately decreased the likelihood that they would choose to exercise.

Here's how this might play out in our own day. It's Wednesday, and you have nonstop meetings in which you have to think a lot and perform well. The meetings are running late, so you end up grabbing a snack at your desk instead of taking a full lunch break. But after a couple of bites, you get a call—one of the teams you are managing isn't delivering, and you're going to have to step in quickly and do some damage control before your afternoon round of meetings starts. You take care of business and rush back for the next meeting, immediately getting embroiled in a problem-solving discussion. Suddenly, you look at the clock and realize that your day got away from you and it's almost time for that weight-lifting class you just signed up for. Thankfully, the meeting ends. But after a day of intense mental effort, you're drained. It's just too much effort to push through the exhaustion to get to the strenuous exercise on the other side.

Decades of research and years (if not decades) of our own experiences show that what we intend to do is very different than what we actually do.[10] How many times have we resolved to eat less, exercise more, or make more "me" time, only to stumble and fall off the wagon with a forbidden food, a missed class, or the priority of someone else's needs? The reasons are many—family responsibilities, social commitments, conflicting obligations, or activities that are just more fun—but the result is the same. This common phenomenon is referred to as the *gap* between our intentions and behavior. We keep intending and starting, and then we quickly fall down, whether through temptation, rebelling against our own plans, or simply being too tired or confused about which choices to choose.

This gap is not a reflection of our personal failings. In chaotic environments, the rules and standards of behavior change that we've learned—do what your doctor says, hit the target goal, just start anew, form an automatic habit, follow the plan no matter what—add to the static with guilt and confusion. It's hard to figure out what to do next, let alone stick to your eating or exercise program. When we step up the complexity of a task, things get harder. Whether it's something as relatively simple as figuring out how you're going to entertain a visiting friend you haven't seen in years, or something larger and more stressful like suddenly having to move out of your home and sorting out where you're going to live, that demands executive functioning. As Joel Nigg, PhD, professor of psychiatry and director of the Center for ADHD Research at Oregon Health & Science University, explains, "Now imagine having four such problems all at once, and you can see that your capacity would be overwhelmed."[11]

Importantly, and luckily for us, *our executive functioning is activated right when we need it*. It kicks in *when we encounter* novel, unforeseen circumstances to help us analyze and improvise in the moment.[12] It is executive functioning that allows us to solve the unforeseen problems thrown up by the many small and large challenges to our daily plans: a canceled appointment that gives us three hours to fill, a sudden downpour that puts the damper on a planned picnic, a roadwork detour that causes us to figure out a new route to our destination.

Executive functioning helps us sort through our choices and priorities in the moment and make a new plan that suits the new circumstances. It does this primarily through three cognitive abilities: working memory, mental flexibility, and inhibition. We'll explore the truly awesome nature of our executive functioning a little later in this book, and learn the fun, simple, and science-based strategies designed to support them so they can do what they are designed to do: help us make the in-the-moment choices that keep us *consistent and on track with our greater goals* (in our case, around healthy eating and exercise), goals that align with our core values to serve not only our own needs but the needs of the people and things we most value.[13]

But hold that thought—we'll get to those strategies in the second part of this book. Right now, the next chapter begins our exploration of the hidden but powerful forces that keep us from achieving lasting change, and dives into the common decision disruptors that so often trap our best intentions.

three

WHY WE DON'T "JUST DO IT"

N 2017, NOBEL PRIZE–WINNING PSYCHOLOGIST AND DECISION MAKING expert Daniel Kahneman was speaking at an academic summit to a group of behavioral scientists. One of these participants asked his advice about how they could help people make behavioral changes they could sustain. Kahneman responded that there is a good way to change behavior and a bad way. The bad way asks, *How can I drive this behavior?* The good way asks instead, *Why aren't I doing it already?* For this group of scientists, this one hit home.

Kahneman explained that he learned this strategy as an undergraduate from pioneering social psychologist Kurt Lewin, and he calls it "the best advice I ever heard in psychology."[1] I have always believed that this is also great advice for anyone who embarks on trying to change a complex behavior like eating or exercise. Lewin's classic, now reemerging *force field* analysis[2] addresses the continual tug-of-war between two opposing forces that act on the in-the-moment decisions that ultimately constitute our behavior: For every choice, there is a *driver* (I need to get healthier) and a *resister* (I have to eat that crème brûlée because it would be rude to turn it down).

Kahneman's advice suggests a radical departure from what we've typically learned about behavior change. Instead of turning up the heat on the driver, trying to motivate ourselves with more cajoling, incentives, and trying to hold them there with the force of our will-power, we need to look at what's *resisting* these healthy choices and disrupting our desired decisions related to better eating and being physically active.

MINDSET OVER MATTER

A lot of popular behavior change trends are built on reducing the resisters that exist outside of ourselves in our *physical environment*. Carefully constructing our daily contexts (avoiding smokers if you're trying to quit smoking) and living spaces to support our lifestyle change (buying a treadmill to use in the basement, tossing the bags of potato chips in the trash) can be important environmental-level strategies. Unfortunately, once we walk out the door of our well-built behavior house, all hell breaks loose.

To understand how this works, consider athletes. As long as athletes are playing their sport, they have external structures and contexts to support their participation: scheduled games, planned practices, coaches' expectations, and a community of fans. But as research shows,[3] many athletes, even passionate ones, do not keep up their regimens once they leave the team or stop playing their sport. This happens because they have not learned the necessary mindset for sustaining a physically active life once they *leave the arena* and resume everyday life.

If even disciplined athletes have trouble staying disciplined, where does this leave us regular folks? The answer takes us right

back to Lewin, who paid special attention to the driving and disrupting forces that exist *within our own mind, at the exact moment* of
choice.[4]

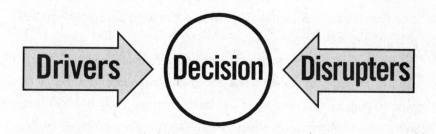

Traditionally, our approaches to eating and exercise have tended
to be logistically focused—what gym to join, which social network
to engage in for camaraderie, what app to buy. These strategies are
concrete and easy to wrap our heads around. We can see and feel
an exercise bike, but our mental phenomena are always just passing
through. Compared to a new smart watch, our thoughts and feelings are all too easy to write off as inconsequential. Yet, according to
Lewin,[5] and the emerging theories about eating[6] and exercise,[7] these
mental phenomena have a strong influence on our momentary decision making. Lewin terms this invisible yet substantial force our "life
space."

Let's take a step back from this conversation and just consider
the term *life space*. I don't know about you, but that term makes me
feel grounded. Just by recognizing my life space as valid I am taking
myself and my emotional and psychological world as seriously as the
physical world. This is *my* life, *my* space. It's real, valid, and important
for me to take into consideration.

Whether we realize it or not, this world of emotions and memories, thoughts and feelings, influences how we interact with the
people, events, and tasks we encounter in daily life, and the choices

we make—including the choices we make about eating and exercise. Just like the continual parade of experiences that play out in our day, our life space is also inherently dynamic. It shifts, transforms, and changes at any point in time based on our internal physical and emotional states as well as our reactions to the external circumstances playing out in our day.

Each of us has our own unique life space. It is composed of our moods, needs, and perceptions about this moment, coupled with how they are influenced not only by our future goals but by all of our past experiences in life, including those involving eating, exercise, and those that are more personal—being a daughter, a son, a partner, a friend, a parent, a student, an employee, a supervisor, an artist, a scientist, a teacher, a businessperson...

As I write this chapter, for example, I am a researcher, a writer, a coach, a mom, a spouse, and a daughter. I didn't get quite enough sleep last night, so I'm also tired and finding it harder than usual to organize my thoughts, which increases my anxieties about finishing this chapter! You may want to take a moment to consider the many *you's* who exist in your life space right now, and how your life space changes (or does not change) from day to day.

Clearly, we are complex beings.

DECISION DISRUPTORS

The beauty of the life space concept is that it values the complex, ever-changing realities we live with inside our minds. It doesn't pretend that we can take a behavioral choice like "get to bed at ten p.m." or "exercise Monday through Friday at five thirty a.m. for half an hour" and isolate it from the hubbub in the rest of our lives. *That very hubbub and its influence on our choices resides in our life space too!* Lewin called out our life space, the space of our *innermost* experiences, as the prime real estate where real change occurs. But it is also the place where our best-laid plans and choices are disrupted.

Every new year brings a new resolution to improve our lives in some way, eat better, get more sleep, exercise, finally take better care of ourselves. But each day also brings something else: a *choice point*—between eating this or that, between going for a walk or continuing to work. And at this choice point, emotional and psychological resisters lurk deep in our life space, trapping us and pulling us away from our plan: You go to work in the morning certain that you'll complete your exercise plan, and *bam!*—you find yourself working till midnight instead. You buy all the ingredients for a meal that fits your eating plan, and *bam!*—you've got a bag of chips in your hand.

I call these powerful forces *decision disruptors*. They feed on the socialization we've had all of our lives, not only about eating and exercise but also about being "good people." This socialization includes the unspoken but real expectations about the "right" way to behave, the specific rules we've been told to follow, the beliefs we hold that come from what our parents teach us, clinicians appointments, our interactions with peers, and the visual and verbal messages we pick up from advertising, news, magazines, and social media. All of these ideas, both conscious and unconscious, powerfully influence our decision making about eating and exercise, often in ways we don't see or understand.

These decision disruptors quite literally disrupt our decisions at the moment of choice, often before we realize it. I've found the following four decision disruptors to be the most common across my clients, and I'm betting at least one of them is a familiar frenemy of yours:

+ **Decision Disruptor #1: TEMPTATION:** *We give in to the easy, tempting choice.* We feel "tempted" by things we feel we shouldn't have or don't deserve yet that we want. Often, our impulses overpower our healthy intentions despite the fact that our more rational self knows that we'll be left feeling guilty and disappointed by our perceived "weakness" or "lack of self-control."

+ **Decision Disruptor #2: REBELLION:** *We triumphantly rebel against "shoulds."* Science shows that there is often a dissonance between the lifestyle goal we strive to achieve and what this goal actually means to our core sense of self. This inner conflict compels the part of ourselves that feels resentful about being controlled to seek freedom. We instinctively rebel against the very choice we had hoped to make, often feeling self-righteous and triumphant but ultimately sabotaging what we really want.

+ **Decision Disruptor #3: ACCOMMODATION:** *We always put the needs of other people and projects before our own.* Whether we do it from a need to get along, to not be considered selfish, or to put productivity above all else, this level of accommodation undercuts our self-care needs. Ironically, when we consistently compromise our own needs, we are left depleted with much less to give.

+ **Decision Disruptor #4: PERFECTION:** *Aiming for the ideal over the real.* Too exhausted to cook a healthy meal? Might as well fill up on Fritos. No time to work out for forty minutes? No workout today. Can't do it right? Don't do it at all. Mounting science shows that this pervasive perfectionistic thinking gets in the way of coming up with creative strategies that could have taken us to our goal. Because most things in life can't be perfect, unrealistic expectations leave us feeling as though we failed, ultimately demotivating us from doing anything at all.

Here's the kicker: *It's not our "fault" when these decision disruptors so easily arise and pull us under.* We are not born with these disruptors intact. They are generated through life experiences, societal expectations, and the rules of behavior change that we've learned to believe, even though many of us have repeatedly tried to follow them and failed. In the next four chapters, we'll take a closer look at how each of these decision disruptors derail our decisions and take us off course. Because they operate in the dark, outside of consciousness, I think you'll find that just bringing them into the daylight and seeing how they work will help you recognize and more easily disempower them when next you meet.

four

DECISION DISRUPTOR #1: TEMPTATION

JOHN DRAGGED HIMSELF UPSTAIRS AND INTO HIS APARTMENT AFTER A long, hot, stressful day at work during which pretty much everything had gone wrong. He knew he should change clothes for the run he and his wife, Laila, had agreed on this morning, but right now the couch was calling to him. The thought of getting even more tired and sweaty than he was now just made him want a cold drink. Feeling slightly guilty, he tossed his keys on the counter, grabbed a beer from the fridge, and flopped down on the couch. *Yes.*

As he reached for the remote, sinking deeper and deeper into the pillows, Laila walked in, ready to go. She took one look at him and shook her head. "What's up, dude?" she asked. "I thought we agreed to go for a run before dinner." She looked mad. John's heart sank. He *really* didn't want to run right now. What he wanted to do was the exact opposite: relax on the couch, drink a beer, and binge-watch old episodes of 24. Yeah, she was definitely ticked at him. But he couldn't move. In his stressed-out state his motivation had dropped to zero, the temptation he felt to stay put was just too powerful to resist, and he found himself giving in to it even though he *really* hated disappointing Laila.

THE TWO SYSTEMS THAT INFLUENCE OUR CHOICES

John's choice to forgo the run may seem straightforward. After all, he was tired and stressed from an intense day of work. Who wouldn't want to just chill on the couch? Like John, we commonly say things like "I'm not motivated" or "I don't have time" to explain why we've dropped a gym membership or an eating plan. These are valid reasons, but they often mask what's driving those choices on a deeper level, where two systems—one reactive, the other reflective—are often in a continual struggle for our attention and choices.[1]

Although they are often discussed as being two separate, standalone systems, newer thinking considers them as dynamically interrelated.[2] Operating in parallel, these systems regulate our thoughts, feelings, and actions, and have a big impact on our eating and exercise choices.[3] Despite their interrelated nature, some of my clients tell me it's useful to think about these systems as distinct and separate when they think about their choices.

As its name suggests, the reactive system acts quickly! This is where our unconscious plays out, automatically influencing our choices and behavior, often without us even realizing it. It's the system where our urges, cravings, and desires are generated, and where automatic habits form.[4] Like a playful and untrained puppy, the reactive system has a constant desire for pleasure and fun, comfort and affection, and little knowledge of rules or interest in following them.

In stark contrast to the lightning speed of the reactive system, the reflective system is slow. I liken this system to a mentor or wise coach. Unlike the impulsive puppy who acts without reflection, this system is like a coach who thinks things through: deliberating, analyzing the potential consequences of each option, and picking the best one even if it means wrestling our urges down in the process.[5]

Neither system is "good" or "bad." Ideally, they work together in our best interests. And while there are many factors that determine which system is more influential on our eating and exercise at any given moment, one thing never changes: Our choices occur in the moment we make them, and a myriad of factors influence that moment. Stress, fatigue, anxiety, overwhelm, sleep deprivation, alcohol…these are among many types of states and situations that influence whether the reactive or reflective system dominates our choice.[6] Most commonly, these factors stack the deck in favor of the impulsive system, and we make the choice that we had really hoped *not* to make.

WHEN TEMPTATION STRIKES

You *know* when temptation strikes. You may call it a guilty pleasure and enjoy it, or you may feel terrible about "giving in." But whatever you do and whatever your temptation is, it's visceral and potent; an irresistible undertow pulling you toward a pleasure that's hard to resist. Temptation is such a relevant and common disruptor to people's eating and exercise choices that emerging science is centrally focused on it, studying the role that our desires, urges, and cravings play in our eating and exercise decisions.

It's important to note that when we talk about temptation in this context, we are *not* talking about addiction. Although there is debate about whether chronically overeating or binging on certain foods crosses over into "addiction," the Temptation decision disruptor does not reflect any physiological issues that potentially relate to addiction.

It's all too easy to find yourself eating your way through a family-size package of Oreos or fall into a social media scroll that goes on into the early morning hours. We make these choices automatically, despite part of us knowing that they go against the very eating, exercise, and sleep-related plans we made and intended to stick to. But the Temptation decision disruptor is all about immediate pleasure. It doesn't *care* about our future goals. That's one reason why it's so easy for Temptation to win at the point of choice between sticking with long-term goals or feeling happy *right now*.

Temptation is the desire to do something, whether it's something we just want, or something that might be considered unwise or forbidden. In its very essence, temptation is (consciously or unconsciously) *emotion remembered*.[7] It becomes the Temptation decision disruptor when it motivates us to act against our intended plans and long-term goals at the point of choice *because of remembered experiences*—whether it's a painful memory of shame in a junior high gym class, or the delightful sensory memory of a cream-filled chocolate éclair.

The new emerging theories about eating and exercise have opened up some exciting insights into what's really happening at the point of choice. And that brings us back to the couch with John and his conflict between running with his wife or vegging out for the evening.

UNDERSTANDING THE ART OF EXERCISE

John's dilemma reflects the classic conflict so many of us face between our intentions and goals and our feelings, preferences, and temptations at the exact moment of decision about whether to exercise or not. This specific instance of momentary conflict is so pervasive around the world that Ralf Brand and Panteleimon Ekkekakis devised the Affective–Reflective Theory (ART) of physical inactivity and exercise to explain it.[8]

According to the ART, we need to consider John's decision as occurring within the context of the specific moment. *Right now*, John is exhausted and stressed. *Right now*, he is sinking happily into his couch. *Right now*, he is also recalling his intention to go for a run with his wife. He *knows* this would be valuable for both his health and his relationship, but the mere thought of exercise gives him an uneasy *feeling*.

Leaps and bounds beyond the traditional thinking related to how to motivate people to exercise, the ART is based on a dual-process model—the two processes reflecting the two systems we just discussed, the reactive (affective, feeling) system and the reflective (logical thinking) system. It is designed to explain the psychological mechanisms underlying the *situated decisions* (the decisions we make in a specific moment) in which we face dilemmas about whether to exercise or blow it off.

The ART's fundamental proposition is that for many people the idea of exercising has been associated with an unpleasant stew of pain, discomfort, and displeasure. Whether from a shaming experience as a child or teen, inept feelings during a more recent visit to the gym, or feeling uncomfortable when exercising due to carrying extra body weight, the ART contends that these distressing experiences "tag" or brand exercising in negative ways. And like other visceral factors, such as fatigue, pain, and exhaustion from exercising, they are aversive and decrease the desirability of doing it. These negative tags create memories that are considered implicit (unconscious), creating a gut feeling of distaste or disdain that strongly influences our subsequent conscious thoughts about exercising.[9]

Because this gut feeling is the result of our past exercise experiences, it arises spontaneously at the moment of choice. And because

it is from the reactive system, it's automatic: we can't control its arising. This mental shortcut easily bypasses the goals and plans of the
reflective system, pushing us to remain reclining on our comfy couch,
just like John.

The ART supports what I've seen with most of my clients. If
you have had similar negative experiences with exercising, these ideas
might have struck a chord with you as well. If so, when you face a
similar conflict and feel tempted in that moment to remain inactive,
consider this: What might be going on beneath the surface that's
driving you *away from* exercise and *toward* the couch?

THE POWER OF MEMORY

You are passing by your favorite café, vaguely proud of yourself for
having eaten a sensible breakfast, when your eyes are drawn to the
pastry display. The freshly baked fruit tarts and chocolate croissants
are glistening like jewels in the window and stopping you in your
tracks. The door is closed, but even so, you would swear you can smell
the aroma and even feel the butter-rich confections melting in your
mouth, and you remember laughing with your friend the last time
you were together at the café before work. Suddenly, you're starving.
Without thinking, this full-body feeling of sensory happiness carries
you through the door, into the café, and waiting in line to place your
order.

As you no doubt know, when it comes to the Temptation decision disruptor, it's not just exercise we're talking about. Scientific
advances have given us an increased understanding of how the brain
makes decisions, and new thinking helps us learn what's going on
behind the scenes when we are in the process of succumbing to that
tempting treat. And you may not be surprised to discover that memory plays a massive role in what happens here too.

As the ART does with exercise, the *grounded-cognition theory of desire* proposes that our eating experiences create rich situated memories.[10] And they don't use the word "rich" lightly: any memory from a single eating episode includes an abundance of different information, including visual and sensory (what the food or drink item looks like, tastes like, its texture), social and contextual (who else was present, time of day, place), motor (chewing, cutting, swallowing), and our current state (such as our level of hunger and pleasure). That's a lot to bring to a choice point about whether to eat a chocolate croissant!

The researchers explain that our knowledge (that is, our *cognition*) related to eating choices is *grounded* by nonconscious simulations of the relevant senses that are involved when we eat, such as taste and vision, and these cultivate desire toward eating. Below the seemingly straightforward act of reaching for a tempting treat lies a powerful matrix of memories and experiences. Walking by the café cues our minds to create vivid simulations: the feel of a frothy latte; eating the croissant, reexperiencing its chocolate taste and warm, creamy texture, picking it up and putting it into our mouth, and chewing it. These simulations in our mind, grounded in our past experience, generate real desire and feelings of anticipation, creating the raw experience of temptation.

It probably won't surprise you to learn that these types of sensory stimulations based on past eating experiences happen all day long[11]— in the office, at the grocery store, at parties, and even in our own pantries. They contribute to our desires and to giving in to temptation, *especially* for the foods and drink we perceive as especially tasty and enjoyable.[12] In fact, even just *viewing* food images during a brain scan activates the very same brain areas that are involved in actual eating, such as taste, motor, and reward areas.[13]

The way we frame particular foods can be powerful. One study on this idea[14] gave two groups of participants the exact same soup, but described it to one group as "rich and delicious" while telling the other group they were going to drink "boiled vegetable water." Would you be surprised to learn that the group given the label presenting the solution as delicious rated it as tasting better compared to the group given "boiled vegetable water"? Probably not. The effect from putting a simple frame around what we are about to eat and drink is simple, swift acting, and even visible: The neuroimaging research showed that the "rich and delicious" group participants showed stronger associated reward activations in the brain compared to the group told it was boiled veggie water.

More recent research supports this finding by showing that framing veggie dishes with sensory-focused terms (such as "Sweet Sizzlin' Green Beans and Crispy Shallots") increased consumers' taste ratings and choices compared to health-focused terms (such as "Light 'n Low-Carb Green Beans and Crispy Shallots").[15] Even though we might not be conscious of it happening, seeing "healthy" labels for foods may simulate a past negative eating experience, such as eating food low in salt that wasn't so tasty; and these memories impact our current eating perceptions and experiences of other "healthy" foods.

Here's the takeaway: The moment we encounter a cue for or even just think about something delicious, a rich neuro network of sensory, contextual, and pleasure-based memories is put into action to cultivate desire and make falling to temptation more likely. So, the next time someone suggests that you "just need more self-control," by all means, remind yourself that "control" has very little to do with it. But later in the book, you'll read about new research that discusses how people are learning to successfully navigate feelings of temptation.

TEMPTATION—IT'S COMING FROM INSIDE THE HOUSE

Exercising and eating are two very distinct activities with their own theories and research, but they share a similar underlying phenomenon. Both the ART of physical inactivity and exercise and the eating-focused grounded-cognition theory of desire show us that when it comes to temptation, it's not external but internal, and it's more complex than we're used to thinking.

Temptation goes deep. When you feel tempted to eat another plate of pasta or avoid a workout, that temptation is often related to memories of past experiences—both negative and positive. The cake is just a cake we want, the exercise is just an activity we loathe. But below the surface of our minds, the cake and the activity evoke specific memories and their accompanying feelings and images and sensations, tempting us toward that tasty treat or away from the awful activity.

This might feel overwhelming, but it is very good news. It means that you are not a "lazy" or "gluttonous" person for "giving in to temptation." These forces have been working outside of your awareness and conscious control, and coming to life within your current-day life space. In my coaching work with clients, I have found that when we get the hidden truth about the Temptation decision disruptor out into the open, we can better understand and diminish its powerful pull. Then the next time we are faced with that pastry of our dreams, we can also say "I see you, Temptation!" and tip our hats to a wonderful memory, then move on down the street.

If you are still feeling a little overwhelmed by the power of our unconscious memories to influence both eating and exercise choices, take heart. As you will learn later in this book, we can use our wonderful, elastic brains to *change those memories* into more positive ones that will better keep us on track.

five

DECISION DISRUPTOR #2: REBELLION

S CREW IT, I'M HAVING THE PIZZA!"

That was Lydia's declaration of war against choosing to eat the fat-free, flavor-free vegetable plate from the newest eating rules her doctor had prescribed, and she told me about it defiantly at the beginning of our second session.

If giving in to Temptation makes us feel guilty, rebelling against feeling controlled feels empowering. Eating choices or exercise plans that feel imposed or restrictive predictably create a context where we have no motivation *not* to push back. And, most often, we push back with abandon.

So, Lydia's pizza declaration didn't surprise me. She had already told me about her lifelong struggles with food and eating. Her parents kept what they saw as their "overweight" child on continual diets, and as a self-identified "overweight" adult she had continued that trend for herself—cycling through goals, hope, dieting, weight loss, calorie restriction, rebellion, weight regain…again and again and again. Each new start and subsequent failure amplified her anger and shame. Rebellion, in contrast, felt great.

Quite honestly, I have never read a more perfect portrayal of how Rebellion feels than Catherine Gray's in *The Unexpected Joy of the Ordinary*. Before publication, she asked me to fact-check her description of my research for her soon-to-be best-selling book. Within moments of reading, I burst out laughing. Gray had nailed the rebellious instinct that rears up within our psyches when we believe we *should* exercise in certain ways: "If you find that exercise feels like a chore," she writes, "then it's because you feel like you *should*, rather than you *want to*. Personally, I think the *should* motivation also wakes up our kohl-eyed teenage anarchist, who wants to give *what we should do* the finger and go and smoke weed instead."[1]

That, in essence, is what the Rebellion decision disruptor is all about.

Whatever the source and whatever our age, when our freedom and sense of autonomy feels threatened, our psyche is automatically motivated to react against that which threatens to take it away. We skip the "good for us" vegetables, ignore the digital reminders we've set for ourselves, ditch the exercise class that pushes us too hard. *Whatever* it takes to reclaim our sense of autonomy.

Contrary to the typical behavior change story we've been told all of our lives, eating the pizza when we had intended not to isn't really about our lack of self-control. Often, it instead reflects an innate drive to reclaim our right to personal choice when *shoulds*—in Lydia's case, the belief that she should stay on her diet no matter what, that she should absolutely not eat a high-calorie food like pizza—threaten that freedom. Unfortunately, in our society, the *shoulds* are all around us.

THE *SHOULDS* WE LIVE WITH

Get plenty of sleep! Don't eat carbs! Meditate! Eat more vegetables! Stay in shape!

Even the most positive health promotion communications and methods in our society often feel controlling, sometimes bordering on dogmatic, and perhaps nowhere as much as with eating and exercise where judgment flows like water. We are prescribed the "right" way to exercise, told to eat "good" foods rather than "bad" foods, and urged to take better care of ourselves "or else." The obligatory *shoulds* and directives we are on the receiving end of go on and on. Yet mounting research suggests that the traditional health promotion messaging related to exercise and eating may do more harm than good.

A group of researchers investigated whether they could create a rebellion-like response to a future exercise class, *even when* participants expected it to be fun and enjoyable.[2] Two groups of participants read the same description of the upcoming class, *except that* one group's ad contained autonomy-supporting language that emphasized choice and individual preferences (e.g., "we all feel differently about exercise"), while the other group's ad included controlling language (e.g., "you must do it now," "this exercise class is better than yours"). As hypothesized, the participants who read the controlling messages reported greater rebellion-like responses than those who read the language supporting autonomy, despite both groups' expecting that the exercise class would be fun. Damn!

Some conditions, like uncertainty, can reduce reactance;[3] and some cultures might be less sensitive to having their individual freedom threatened (individualist versus collectivistic).[4] Despite differences like these, prescriptive language commonly used to promote health, better eating, and regular exercise, and other self-care behaviors can generate anger and resentment and motivate Rebellion.[5] And we are just starting to learn that even seemingly innocuous behavioral support and motivation strategies like "nudges" can have similar unintended negative effects.

NUDGE, NUDGE

Nudges—such as nutrition labeling on foods and "take the stairs" signs placed by elevators—are commonplace these days. On websites, nudges are a way to design digital "choice architecture" so that a particular choice becomes more likely based on how it is presented.[6] Nudges have become pervasive across corporate wellness, health, and fitness arenas. As described in a recent session about nudges at an industry conference put on by Omada Health,[7] nudges come in many forms, including economic (such as incentives and rewards like paying an employee to exercise more) or social (such as competitions based on increased health promoting behaviors among a community of people).

The session facilitators, Jennifer La Guardia, PhD, director of Clinical Product and Behavior Science at Omada Health, and Amy Bucher, PhD, VP of Behavior Change Design at Mad*Pow, said that nudges can also be "direct prods, such as push notifications or unsolicited pings or text messages reminding you it's time to get up to exercise, take your medication, or step on the scale."[8] Nudges are designed to gently push people in a certain direction, in theory making those choices more likely; they don't have the power to force people's actions. But like some health promotion language, even gentle nudges have the potential to be experienced as paternalistic or even create a boomerang effect.[9]

Like any simple strategy that aims to influence decisions or change behavior, nudges must be designed intentionally, using the right science that works *with* rather than *against* people's autonomy, momentary needs, and circumstances. Otherwise, nudges that are intended to remind people to make a healthy choice, such as to take a work break in order to exercise, often wind up becoming annoying "noodges" that pressure and nag.[10] And—this is *not* a cliffhanger!— what happens next is that we become annoyed, sometimes even angry. Just as reactance theory predicts what would happen,[11] we can become defiant and motivated to rebel against the nudge, either avoiding or disengaging from our target behavior or even ditching the nagging app entirely.

Michael told me that's exactly what happened to him when he decided to start exercising before a long-delayed summer vacation. His friends were all talking up a hot new exercise app, and he figured it would help him get motivated. He generally hated gyms, and that's where the activity seemed to be. But this app gave you workouts you could do with or without home equipment. It not only kept track of your stats and progress, but reminded you when it was time to work out and for how long.

The first two days, he loved it. The goals were clear, the graphics were great, and the interface was intuitive and friendly. He felt in control of his program. But by day three, the pings reminding him that he hadn't completed (or started) an activity were starting to annoy him, especially when they went off in the middle of something else he was doing. This app had its own agenda, and it wasn't Michael's. For Michael, the pings never stopped feeling like an unwelcome poke in the ribs. He couldn't just ignore it, so he triumphantly deleted the app.

IT FEELS SO *GOOD*

Here's a sentence I've heard from *many* clients. They come home after a hard day of work, reach for a "forbidden" food—a bag of chips, a pint of ice cream, an entire pizza—and eat all of it, saying to themselves, "Dammit, I deserve it!"

Rebellion—even against our own carefully made plans—is a powerful, energizing force. It can feel like a dangerous *thrill*. More exciting than doing the forty minutes of exercise you signed up for, more fun than eating the greens you bought for dinner, and that your doctor says are good for you, more enticing than going to bed and getting enough sleep to work more efficiently the next day. The Rebellion decision disruptor is like your inner toddler (or teenager) coming out and saying, *You can't make me!* Unfortunately, that "you" is also *you* and *your* self-selected plans and good intentions.

So, why do we rebel, seemingly, against ourselves?

Because it is an innate human response to feel rebellious defiance toward feeling pressured or dominated. Formally called *reactance*, Rebellion refers to the drive we experience to reclaim our freedom when we feel that we are being controlled.[12] Under the right circumstances, Rebellion is a healthy choice: it helps us protect our self-determination and can keep us alive in the most dire circumstances. This inclination is lifesaving if you're being held captive. But the problem with Rebellion is that it also flips on at the most mundane times, as in this familiar exchange:

"Eat your broccoli, Robert, it's good for you."

"I won't eat it, and you can't make me!"

Whichever side of that discussion you might be on (and maybe you've been on both sides at different points in your life), I bet you understand this dynamic. We accept this rebellious stance toward healthy eating as a natural part of the turbulent toddler or teenage years, when young people are developing and learning to express their autonomy. But, as Lydia's example shows, in our society individualism is prized, and Rebellion is not "just a phase." It's alive and well as long as we are.

WHEN MINDS COLLIDE

Fighting the good fight against the *shoulds* is just one type of Rebellion. Another type of Rebellion motivates us to stand up to an even more oppressive dynamic: a divided self that believes *yes, I can* while chanting *no, you can't* at the same time. This Rebellion is more profound and commonly experienced among those of us who have struggled with our weight for much of our lives. This *cognitive dissonance*[13]—a fight between two conflicting beliefs, values, or states—motivates us to reduce the discrepancies that make us feel uncomfortable.

Feeling cognitive dissonance is not only mentally exhausting, it is problematic for many other reasons. The obvious one is that it often undermines the exercise and eating plans we make for ourselves. But more fundamentally, cognitive dissonance conflicts with our innate human need for self-determination. It undermines our need to align our beliefs and actions with our core sense of self and the internal sense of coherence, well-being, and consistency that brings.[14]

Let's dig deeper into how feeling a discrepancy between these two selves thwarts our eating and exercise plans. Beyond a basic reactance against the thought, *I should eat that bland vegetable plate on my diet because Dr. Thompson told me to*, is a whole lot of past experience: the voices of negative judgments about our weight that we've heard all our life. That's a lot to carry in your head every time you're faced with a challenging food choice.

I asked Jennifer Taber, PhD, social psychologist in the Department of Psychological Sciences at Kent State University, who conducts research on reactance to health information, about the personal decision making that tries to lessen cognitive dissonance.[15] She started with the common example of how it works with smoking. "Smokers," she explained, "are a classic example of people who experience cognitive dissonance. If people believe smoking is bad for their health but they continue to smoke, then they have cognitive dissonance around smoking. And to reduce it, they either have to quit smoking—which is really hard—or change their cognitions about smoking, by starting to believe, for example, that it's not that bad or making a plan to quit at some vague time in the future." But she also discussed how cognitive dissonance could play out with eating. She said that when people are conflicted in the way my client was, they can temporarily reduce their dissonance around a food choice by rebelling, and eating something that flies in the face of the healthy eating plan they had created for themselves.

When we eat the forbidden food to push back against the "rules," we might be trying to reduce the cognitive dissonance between these two divergent parts of ourselves. Although any momentary rebellion is not sufficient to resolve a cognitive dissonance that reflects a lifelong struggle, for Lydia, eating the pizza—in that moment—represented one way she could align with her positive self-worth and agency. I can't tell you how common this phenomenon is, especially for women. Most of my female clients tell me they resonate with this phenomenon on some level, and I myself have lived this painful inner divide at certain points of my life.

The social stigma that accompanies being considered "fat," "out of shape," "not muscular enough," or simply not fitting with society's vision of the "ideal" body type or physical abilities can be crushing. Just writing about it doesn't do it justice to the full-bodied, mind-harming, empirically documented devastation it can cause. Weight bias and its accompanying stigma results in increasing vulnerability to stress, depression, low self-esteem, poor body image, maladaptive eating behaviors, and avoidance of physical activity.[16]

Socialization and stigma might be hard for some to see but it is ever-present for many others. We breathe it like air, take it into our cells, and it becomes part of who we are, our sense of ourselves and our self-worth. Studies show that when we carry more weight, the weight bias and negative judgment we receive gets under our skin in the most literal sense: we actually internalize and *embody* these negative judgments toward ourselves and aggression toward our own bodies.[17] And because the observer's perspective that we internalize is one of hostility and degradation, it creates a cognitive dissonance about our sense of self that divides us between feelings of self-worth and self-degradation, putting us at war with our bodies and ultimately with ourselves. Social media, with apps like Facetune and filters that enable us to eliminate so-called imperfections, only increases our insecurities with how we look to others, and amplifies the belief that we don't measure up. Research suggests that simply *perceiving* ourselves as overweight is associated with poorer health.[18]

Unfortunately, what has also happened in our culture is that physical activity and healthy eating have gotten all tangled up in the classic *shoulds* related to weight and health, and the associated stigma and shame. This entanglement is a core reason so many of us experience cognitive dissonance about what should *really be* just great choices to take care of ourselves. This cognitive dissonance about eating and exercise goes beyond simply undermining the potential for productive conversations in clinician counseling and positive experiences at gym visits. It creates a continual inner tug-of-war about food and movement choices when we are at home. We might feel triumphant in the moment of seemingly reclaiming our freedom to choose, but shortly afterward, we find ourselves feeling on empty. And while this phenomenon is so pervasive, because shame is involved, many, especially women, assume they are alone and at fault, which further deepens the pain.

The cognitive dissonance we experience about this topic is completely different from the commonly discussed conflict that occurs between our logical, future-oriented goals and our impulsive right-now desires and temptations, respectively. In this case, it's not about whether our impulses or logic will win. Instead, it's about the conflict between our real desire to take good care of ourselves with that "good" food choice and our want to give that choice the finger.

With such potent *shoulds* as the cultural backdrop, it's no surprise that people who exercise for weight-related reasons tend to be less committed, feel more controlled about exercising, and participate less than people who are active to enhance their daily sense of well-being.[19] Think about it: shame, rebellion, and dissonance take up space in our mind, as do the negative memories about our old experiences with eating and exercise that we carry with us. These forces and energies constrict and contract our thinking. They create noise and take up space, depleting our energy and mental resources and undermining the very executive functioning we need to make the choice that, deep down, *we* really want to make.

So, was Lydia's choice to eat the pizza purely unproductive and self-defeating, another failure on her diet journey, as you might have previously believed? Given all that we now understand about reactance, our urge to regain control of our own lives, the crushing power of weight bias, and the confusion of cognitive dissonance, her Rebellion could be considered not as self-sabotage, but as an act of self-affirmation.

No, I am not suggesting Rebellion as a remedy. It's also important to remember that because our rebellion is in direct reactance to the *shoulds*, the irony is that we are still being controlled by the very thing we are rebelling against. Real solutions to this systemic problem need cultural level change.[20] But as individuals, we have no choice but to also grapple with these feelings and choices and the specific lifestyle goals they may be connected to.

Understanding the complexity of these issues and tempering our actions with self-compassion is an important step toward achieving the eating and exercise success we are after. As we begin to understand our decision disruptors like Rebellion and how they work, we are readying ourselves to recognize them at our choice points and let them go so we can finally see the *alternative* options that are all around us.

six

DECISION DISRUPTOR #3: ACCOMMODATION

S TEPHANIE, HER HUSBAND, AND THEIR TWO TEENAGERS WERE ENJOYING their annual weekend at a beach house with two other families they had become friends with when their kids were in preschool. The families had been eagerly awaiting this time to be together, and they had each contributed a dish to their traditional celebratory Sunday feast.

It was a noisy, fun-filled meal with lots of laughter. But at dessert, things got a little sticky for Stephanie when her friend brought forth a beautiful three-layer cake she had baked especially for the occasion. For the last four months, Stephanie had been committed to a new eating plan, and chocolate cake was not on it. While she was still surprised by it, her more mindful eating had reduced the intense cravings for dessert she used to have. Yet she has a very hard time saying no, especially in social settings.

From our conversations, I knew she had been feeling really great about her new way of eating. She had come to our coaching deeply committed to making this change, and after four months she was going strong. I had witnessed her transformation: from being rebellious about "having to make" different eating choices, to a deep sense of ownership and satisfaction that embodied the type of self-determination that is thought to be important for cultivating long-term behavior change.[1] So, when the cake arrived, neither Temptation nor Rebellion were calling to her.

But something else just as powerful *was* staring her down in that moment. For Stephanie, not having dessert at this event was more complicated than turning down cake. On a deeper level, it meant that she was not meeting the needs of people she deeply cared about. Just the thought of bursting the communal cake bubble evoked feelings of selfishness and guilt. So, despite not being hungry or even *wanting* the cake, Stephanie smiled and accepted a big slice to accommodate what she perceived to be the celebratory needs of the group.

Eating the cake didn't lead Stephanie to abandon her new eating routine altogether, but it didn't make her feel great about herself either. She was happy that she didn't make waves during the celebration, or have to deal with explaining to her friend why she was refusing something her friend had clearly worked hard to prepare. But she didn't really enjoy it, and she didn't enjoy the feeling that she had let herself down.

IS ACCOMMODATION ALTRUISM?

When I was thinking about what to name this very common decision disruptor, *altruism* was on the table. Altruism is defined as the practice of unselfish concern for or devotion to the welfare of others.[2] And that definitely sounds like Stephanie! She *is* very concerned with the well-being and welfare of others. But the phenomenon at play that night wasn't really about altruism, it was about something else: accommodating the needs of others to the exclusion of her own. Accommodating is generally a positive term, and certainly it can be a lovely thing to do. But even the best things are better in moderation. When we *always* sacrifice our own self-care needs for those of others, accommodation crosses over from being a virtue to being the Accommodation decision disruptor.

It's also important to point out that Stephanie's choice to eat the cake was not based on a decision to be flexible with her eating plan so she could partake in the festivities. A decision that would have reflected a type of flexible restraint that actually is considered an *adaptive eating strategy*.[3] Stephanie ate her cake and made the requisite sounds of enjoyment, but her choice was the opposite of celebratory.

Later, she admitted to me (and to herself) that her choice to eat the cake reflected a long-term pattern to meet the needs of others by sacrificing her own. And it was not so much a choice as a grudging decision that left her feeling diminished, like she had lost a part of herself, less whole and competent than she had felt before the meal. For days afterward, negative self-judgment became her constant companion. And predictably, this self-indicting rumination was accompanied by a low mood and comfort eating, spiraling her into the desert of discouragement—nowhere near the land of empowered eating and self-motivated self-care she had lived in for the past four months.

This story may sound dramatic, a huge outcome for such a seemingly trivial choice, but it is a true story and it happens all the time in the context of eating, exercise, and other self-care behaviors. The Accommodation decision disruptor doesn't just nibble at our intended eating and exercise choices; it can feel like a wave that builds up a force so great that, like Stephanie, we feel washed away.

So, no, it is not altruism, and it's not just "being a nice person." Rather, the Accommodation trap that some of my clients fall into

reflects a profound disregard of our own self-care needs. And ironically, this seemingly selfless decision can have unforeseen negative
consequences for the very people we thought we were serving.

THE BURNOUT RISK OF SELFLESS GIVING

Like many of my clients, Stephanie falls into the classic "giver" cat-
egory. Givers are frequently motivated by the desire to protect and
promote the well-being of others.[4] Wharton organizational psychologist and best-selling author Adam Grant established the counterintuitive notion that "givers," people who are other focused and care
about contributing to and supporting others and their endeavors,
frequently reap the rewards of their altruism by achieving success
across numerous life areas. In addition, when we give, our health and
well-being benefit.[5] Givers embody prosocial traits, such as selfless-
ness, altruism, and kindness; and in this context, it's hard to argue
that being a giver is anything but great. But there is a subgroup of
givers who don't fare so well.

These *selfless givers* sacrifice *too* much. They are overly accommodating to others at the expense of their own energy.[6] Selfless givers
are inclined to drop everything when people need something from
them. They exemplify what's called *unmitigated communion,* "a focus
on and involvement with others to the exclusion of the self,"[7] and
pathological altruism, "a need to sacrifice oneself for the benefit of others."[8] People who fall into these categories usually agree with statements like "I always place the needs of others above my own," "I am
a total pushover when it comes to requests for help," "I often feel run
down due to the demands of others," or "Even when exhausted, I will
always help other people."

Certainly, it is important to tend to the needs of others, even if it
means we sometimes have to subsume our own. This is something a

parent learns early on and some cultures value this more than others. But with a little distance it also becomes clear that generally agreeing with these statements easily puts us at risk of consistently neglecting our *own* self-care, something research shows is associated with depression, anxiety, distress, and poor health behaviors—and even worse health outcomes related to diabetes.[9]

Clearly, when there is an imbalance between the care and concern we give to others and to ourselves, we are at a higher risk for burnout and getting sick. These are high stakes. The irony that Grant points out is that more than thirty years of data, across many metrics, show that the most selfless givers actually give *less* than givers who balance concern for others with concern for the self. "If you are selfless to the point of self-sacrifice, at some point you run out of energy and resources to be able to contribute to others."[10]

THE SELFLESS LEADER

Bryan, the director of family medicine at a progressive health system, heard me speak at a conference about the intersection of clinician and patient self-care and asked me to help his team. He invited me to deliver an all-day training on how to coach patients about healthy eating and exercise in ways that will better promote engagement, buy-in, and behavioral sustainability. Bryan had scheduled the training to occur soon after the new family medicine clinic had been built. It was a state-of-the-art health-care facility that also included a full-service gym that was free for all staff members. This fit with the positive assumptions I had made about him as a health leader, and as a person strongly committed to healthy lifestyles and self-care. So, what happened at the end of that day took me completely by surprise.

After the training, as I was speaking with some attendees, Bryan caught my eye and pulled me aside. He seemed to have something urgent to tell me, and he seemed a bit embarrassed. "I have a confession," he said quietly, looking around to make sure no one could hear. Despite being in a profession centered on better health, despite his organization having invested in a gym for everyone to use, and despite being the leader of the clinic, *he did not feel comfortable regularly working out in the gym.* "Why not?" I asked, confused. Bryan confided that his never-ending and ever-growing list of things he needed to do for work always felt more important than exercising.

Can you see where this is heading?

Bryan then confessed that at the few times when he did choose to go to the gym during lunch time, *he tried to hide behind the pillars that lined the hallway to the gym so no one would see that he had stopped working to work out.*

Yup, it's true. But let's be clear about something. It's not that Bryan didn't value the benefits of exercising. He did, and quite strongly. Yet even though he was the boss, and had no one to answer to in his clinic but himself, he still felt the need to cover up his own self-care as almost shameful. You may find this astounding, as I did, or you may easily relate to his plight. Regardless of how you feel, however, the potential impact of Bryan's actions might still surprise you: Research suggests that the consequences of leaders publicly sacrificing their own self-care needs to accommodate their work needs not only hurts their own health, it has a negative effect on the health of the organization as a whole.

TRICKLE-DOWN ACCOMMODATION

One study that investigated the impact of organizational leaders' sleep behavior and messaging on employees highlights just what is at stake. This study of more than six hundred participants from a broad variety of contexts collected data on leader and employee sleep.[11]

Leaders' sleep was assessed with items like "My supervisor talks about getting by with very little sleep" and "My supervisor sends out messages at times when most other people with his/her schedule would be asleep." The findings? When leaders publicly devalue their own sleep, their employees report worse sleep outcomes.

But this study illuminated another negative, and somewhat surprising, finding: Leaders who devalued their sleep, compared to leaders who didn't, rated their subordinates as less likely to act in ethical ways! I spoke with study coauthor Gretchen Spreitzer, PhD, professor of business administration at the University of Michigan's Ross School of Business, to try to understand more about this unexpected finding. She explained that leaders who don't get enough sleep might view their employees with less tolerance, but she also noted other research suggesting that these employees might act less ethically *because of* the organizational culture or simply because they are tired and making poor choices.[12]

It may be that leaders who publicly devalue their own sleep ostensibly signal to employees that loyalty to the organizational culture requires that they, too, should sacrifice sleep for work.[13] Whether out of resentment, payback, or something else, this study and other related research[14] suggests that leaders' public display of devaluing healthy choices like sleep goes beyond simply being a leader's personal preference and cultural norm to a real employee hazard and organizational liability.

We can't know whether anyone else actually saw Bryan hiding behind the pillars in his workout attire, and if they did, whether they interpreted that confusing sight as an explicit signal that, at their clinic, taking time to exercise is really a no-no, despite the new gym. Regardless, I'd wager that staff members are fully aware that Bryan is singularly focused on work, even working through lunch, and that they can't remember ever seeing him at the gym. I'd also wager that many of them also feel guilty about fitting in their own workouts.

PUTTING OUR OWN PRIORITIES LAST?

I've seen it across clients and even in my research. In one study investigating priorities and exercise,[15] we learned a lot from our participants, but one thing that really stood out to us was what participants did *not* discuss: their own self-care. Only one participant in our whole study mentioned where she prioritized herself, noting that, for her, physical activity ranks low because she prioritizes herself and her own needs *at the bottom.*

Whew! I know that sentiment resonates with many people, whether or not they identify it consciously, as this participant did. I've also learned over the years that many people feel somewhat uncomfortable, or sometimes even offended, by the suggestion that there might be any problem with the desire or tendency to strive to accommodate the needs of others, even if it means always sacrificing your own. I'm no longer surprised by this response.

Accommodation, unlike the other decision disruptors, can touch us where we are most vulnerable, in relationship to our undeniable value of and responsibility to care for and nurture family, friendships, relationships, and work. But when we only hear the echo of the word *selfish* when we think about self-care, we are deep in the weeds of Accommodation. As we've seen, there's real science about the damage that can occur when our automatic and consistent go-to is giving other people's needs priority over our own. As with most things in life, seeking balance and finding compromise is key.

The notion that tending to ourselves is simultaneously good for others was made clear during the pandemic. *New York Times* "Well" columnist Tara Parker Pope puts this wisdom into our current day: "The pandemic taught us that when you take care of yourself, you're also taking care of your family, friends and community."[16] Real self-care is anything *but* selfish.

This winning strategy, which we will learn how to implement in the final section of this book, is the one that helps you easily sort through the competing needs of *this* moment to find the creative compromise that allows you to best care for yourself and other people and projects at the same time.

seven

DECISION DISRUPTOR #4: PERFECTION

BEFORE I COULD EVEN GET OUT MY "HELLO," KATY RUSHED INTO TELLING me about her past week of *failed* exercise. Her voice showed a mix of devastation and sheepishness. She was sheepish because she already knew my concerns about her (overly) ambitious weekly goal setting: biking for an hour every day after work and going to the gym before breakfast on Saturday *and* Sunday for a two-hour marathon session. And even though she *knew* her plan wasn't anywhere close to realistic, she still felt devastated that she hadn't even come close to achieving her grandiose goal for the week.

Katy's story was one I had heard many times, and one I continue to hear. It might be the most common tale of frustration with eating and exercise goals, and it's one that has deep roots in the fairy tales we've been told since we were children about what successful eating and exercise looks like.

THE PERFECTION BACKSTORY

Before I took Katy on as a client, she had been reaching out to me for over a year. In her first message to me, which arrived shortly after the New Year, she inquired about becoming a client and also told me exactly what was on her mind: "It's already Jan 28th and my goal to lose 20 pounds and get back in shape has gone nowhere." I informed her that I wasn't taking any new clients then, but we agreed that she would follow up every few months to ask about an opening. While I truly didn't have any openings when Katy contacted me, I also had reservations about working with her.

In the messages that followed she shared her barriers, things like "I don't have enough self-control to work out like the people I follow on Instagram," and "I seem to always put off exercising, I think I'm too lazy." These sentiments are not unique to Katy. But while they reflect current-day conventional thinking, they also reflect what are formally called "exercise-related cognitive errors,"[1] ways of thinking about exercise that are associated with *not* exercising.[2] Above all, her emails raised red flags about working with her; her beliefs showed unrealistic ideals that looked like they might be too entrenched to unearth and change. But despite these misgivings, and because of her tenacious follow-up, I agreed to take her on as a client one year later.

DOWN THE PERFECTION RABBIT HOLE

A key step in my coaching process involves helping clients learn to shift away from the perfectionistic exercise and eating beliefs that, while still widely believed, are now very outdated. In our first session, Katy learned about the recent tectonic shift in exercise recommendations that democratized movement, beginning in 2018 with the publication of the US Department of Health and Human Services' second edition of the *Physical Activity Guidelines for Americans*[3] and culminated with the release of the *World Health Organization 2020 Guidelines on Physical Activity and Sedentary Behaviour*.[4] These new recommendations generally expanded the previous prescription-based requirements targeting specific thresholds of intensity (intensities that cause heavy breathing and sweating) and specific durations (for at least ten minutes but ideally longer) with guidelines emphasizing that *all movement counts*, hoping to inspire people to *choose to move at any and every opportunity that can be created*.

These major changes were not made casually; they were based on updated research about the physical and mental health benefits of physical activity and about how to more successfully help people become and remain *consistently* active. These changed recommendations were accompanied by new scientifically supported campaigns around the world. There was the "Move Your Way" campaign in the United States,[5] the "This Girl Can" campaign in the United Kingdom,[6] and "Follow the Whistle: Physical Activity Is Calling You" (Siga o assobio: *A atividade física chama por si*) campaign in Portugal.[7] The rallying cry from the international community encouraged countries to educate their populations that "Everything counts,"[8] aiming to cultivate a more flexible exercise mindset across the globe.

Because the greater flexibility of these guidelines is so radically different from the past, rigid-by-design recommendations that most people still believe, some clients take more time than others to accept them as valid. Katy, to my surprise, appeared to buy in when she learned about this fundamental shift and I felt a new promise about our work together.

But things did not go as well as I'd hoped. From the start, Katy set weekly exercise goals that were unrealistic, and at the subsequent session she'd berate herself and lament her lack of self-control. When

I suggested that she could be more flexible when barriers arose to her plans, and that there was a myriad of other options to be active on any given day, she dismissed these ideas out of hand.

When we arrived at our fifth session, I decided it was time to address the elephant in the room: Why did she continue to put herself into this same vicious cycle of failure when she had learned about the new, more flexible and forgiving exercise guidelines that give us explicit permission to count all movement as valid and worth doing? Katy explained it to me this way: "Michelle," she said, "I understand the new science and exercise guidelines you told me about. I really heard you, but they don't feel right. What can I say? I just don't want to believe them." And she didn't. Katy didn't show up for our next session, and despite following up with her a few times, I never heard from her again.

This failure was mine, not Katy's. Like most of us, she had internalized this dogmatic exercise ideology from hearing and reading exercise recommendations and messages from the media, the fitness industry, and health care *for decades*. And like so many of my clients at the beginning of our work, she truly believed she could and should meet those outdated standards, despite learning about the new science-based recommendations and despite never having succeeded with the old ones in all her previous attempts.

PERFECTION: THE REAL STORY

Katy's exercise endeavor had fallen prey to the Perfection decision disruptor. Out of all four decision disruptors, Perfection might be the most common and familiar. I want to make it clear that we're *not* talking about perfectionism, which is more of a personality trait; and we are also not talking about a diagnosis of obsessive-compulsive disorder. What we are dealing with here is more specific: the rigid plans and unrealistic goals we've learned equate success when it comes to our eating and exercise.

Targeting the ideal instead of making plans and strategies that take real daily situations into account reflects Perfection. We aim for a bull's-eye, don't consider any alternatives when conflicts arise, and then when our ideal plan doesn't work, we top it off with self-blame. We've essentially limited our choices to two: winning or losing, succeeding or failing. This cycle keeps us stuck as chronic beginners, always starting fresh with high hopes but feeling like failures soon after.

This *is* the success dogma we've been taught, and if it seems "right" to you, as it does to Katy, that's no surprise. Perfectionistic beliefs about exercise and eating and the goals that constitute "success" come from what we've learned to believe over decades. Even though it's not objectively true, and works for only a few, it has been and continues to be the conventional thinking of our time.

The shining vision of the "perfect" plan and "perfect" health and "perfect" body and "perfect" control over our lives and choices is in our minds every time we encounter an eating or exercise choice. And it recedes further and further away from us every time we reach for it. Ironically, the idea that we need to "get it right" when it comes to eating and exercise dooms many of us to an endless cycle of making a new vow, a new resolution, a new start—only to give up when perfect doesn't happen.

IS IT REALLY ALL OR NOTHING?

When we make ideal-over-real plans regarding eating and exercise, our only option is the all-or-nothing thinking that is the root cause of the Perfection decision disruptor. Called *dichotomous thinking*, this way of seeing our plans and goals, and judging the results, is a form of cognitive rigidity. And while you might be able to relate to this black-and-white thinking, you might not know that this mindset goes beyond the conventional way of thinking about creating healthier lifestyles. It's actually considered a type of *distorted thinking* that easily thwarts our goals. The general takeaway may seem counterintuitive. When we think about food in overly rigid ways, we are more likely to restrain our eating in ways that are *un*sustainable.[9]

But all-or-nothing thinking is an equal-opportunity distortion that also works against our workouts, as I have learned in my consulting within the fitness industry. Fitness industry leader Brent Darden, past president and CEO of the IHRSA–The Global Health & Fitness Association, told me that the "largest surge in gym membership around the world is typically the New Year."[10] Every longtime gym member can predict that classes will swell to twice their size on January 2 and almost as quickly shrink back to normal over the next few weeks.

One organization I worked with was interested in identifying which type of new member attendance patterns would predict long-term retention versus dropping out. They discovered two general patterns: one group of members started off after New Year's coming to the gym to work out four to five days per week, while another group of members worked out only one to two days per week. I bet you can guess which group went the distance and which one didn't.

The gym's stats over the year showed that the new members who started out trying to exercise four to five days per week stopped attending pretty quickly, whereas the other group continued to attend and kept their memberships. While this is a single case study, it reflects similar trends across the fitness industry. This jibes with the research discussed above about eating, and aligns with research showing that fantasies about achieving idealized futures predicts decreased energy and poor achievement.[11] It also reflects how all-or-nothing thinking got Katy nowhere in her exercise endeavor, and shows us how quite easily it defeats our hopes of sustainable success.

Perfection is not just the fourth decision disruptor, it also creates the conditions for the other three. And even though it would seem that Perfection's characteristic all-or-nothing thinking would be a great mental simplifier that would support our overall executive functioning, it is actually the opposite. It stops us in our tracks. Perfection, just like the other decision disruptors, leaves no room for compromise about eating the cookie: It's the whole thing or nothing, leaving Temptation, Rebellion, and Accommodation to fight over the spoils. And just like that, right at a challenging moment, we've fallen into the decision disruptor TRAP again.

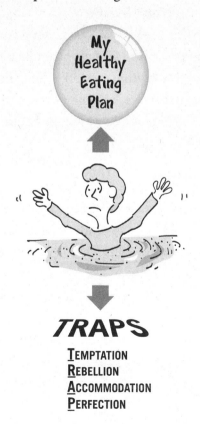

TRAPS

TEMPTATION
REBELLION
ACCOMMODATION
PERFECTION

FALLING INTO THE DECISION DISRUPTORS' TRAP

Temptation, Rebellion, Accommodation, and Perfection. These are our TRAPs.

Rising up, consciously and unconsciously—memories of mouth-watering meals, feeling shamed for adolescent weight problems, being called last for the team in junior high PE, defiance against feeling controlled, feeling selfish about self-care, stressed out by choosing between *the all* or *the nothing*—these disruptors ambush our focus and *trap* our attention, ultimately resisting our hoped-for, planned-for, and well-intended eating or exercise decisions.

But wait: If we had more self-control, couldn't we just over-power *all* of the disruptors? I know we've talked about self-control more than once in this book so far, but it's for a good reason: I can't even count the number of times clients have told me that if they just had more self-control, everything would be fine. Perfection and the need for control are natural companions. So, before we leave Perfection, let's ask one more time: *Don't we just need a little more self-control?*

THE SELF-CONTROL IRONY

The common logic goes like this: If we *just* had enough self-control then we would be able to successfully achieve our (perfectionistic) plans and goals. So, let's dive in a little deeper and see if we can settle the question once and for all.

A set of studies actually looked at this very question, and discovered a surprising answer.[12] Liad Uziel and Roy Baumeister hypothesized that the very state of *wanting* self-control reflects the belief that we don't have *enough* of it (just like Katy told me in her email). In turn, this might stress us out and translate into the belief that we don't have what it takes to succeed.

To investigate this issue, researchers conducted four separate but related studies to look at what happens when people *want to* have more self-control. They asked participants about how much they agreed with statements like "I want to be more self-disciplined" and "I want to be better able to resist temptations," and gave them tasks with differing levels of difficulty or manipulated the desire for more self-control. Across the set of studies, they found that in the face of demanding challenges, simply *desiring to have more self-control* reduced participants' confidence about their abilities to succeed and reduced their performance. The authors contend that *wanting* self-control reflects our worry about being inadequate in the face of challenges, which ironically impairs our performance, demotivates us, and leads us to decide to disengage all together.

Generalizing from this compelling research, *the very belief that if we just had more self-control, we would be successful with our eating or exercise* is taking us in *exactly the wrong direction*: It keeps us shackled by perfectionistic thinking and distracts us from the real solution. Believing we need more self-control puts our attention on perceived inadequacies, reducing our confidence, thwarting our intended eating and exercise decisions, and pretty quickly we ask ourselves, *Why bother?* And we don't.

But the real problem isn't with self-control. It's simply how we've been thinking about it.

THINKING OUTSIDE THE PERFECTION BOX

We've been taught that exerting self-control is the ultimate way to deliver the "perfect" outcomes we're after. But self-control is not designed to be the stand-alone savior, doing all the heavy lifting of behavior change—yet that's how we've learned to see it.

When we're inside the Perfection box, "success" with eating and exercise can mean only one thing: Do it *exactly* right or not at all, hit the impossibly narrow target, right on the bull's-eye. This classic way of thinking isn't just a nonstarter, it is a decision derailer that is also often *in*compatible with our true needs *in the moment*. And over time, what doesn't work in the moment doesn't happen in our lives.

Believing that we need more self-control to succeed only reinforces our belief that we don't have what it takes to get there. And when we fantasize about achieving an idealized outcome in the future (a description of Perfection if I ever heard one), we deplete the energy we need to get there and are subsequently less successful achieving it.

So, if Perfection is truly out of reach, and even reaching for it sets us up to fail, then where do we go from here? We take ourselves outside of the Perfection box and return to the real world, where we will always live amid continual static and interruptions of daily life— the curveballs of unexpected schedule changes, illnesses, mechanical breakdowns, urgent deadlines, and even the happier challenges of celebrations and vacations and falling in love.

Most of us can't succeed at "perfect," but we can succeed at a completely different mindset that is ready and waiting and actually designed to work within the hubbub of our lives: the Joy Choice. The Joy Choice solution is designed to strengthen and support our executive functioning for better eating and regular physical activity. When performing together in an elegant partnership, working memory, flexible thinking, and inhibition can help us calm the overwhelm, sort through the noise, and make the creative compromise—the perfect *imperfect* option—that will guide us to the ever-evolving sweet spot of lasting change.

eight

THE JOY CHOICE: THE PERFECT *IMPERFECT* OPTION

THE OTHER DAY, ONE OF MY FRIENDS MADE AN OFFHAND COMMENT THAT really grabbed my attention. She'd been having conflict after conflict with her preteen daughter, and she was feeling angry, frustrated, and emotionally exhausted. "I know it's not just her, and it's not just her age," she said. "I can think of plenty of things I've said to her in the past that I wish I could take back. Sometimes I feel like I just want to give up!" Then, she laughed and rolled her eyes to let me know she wasn't serious. But it got me thinking.

Like most parents, every day we discover (again) that we can't come close to parenting perfectly. It can be painful when things don't go well, as it is when we belatedly realize that we missed a golden opportunity that our kids were giving us to connect with them about something they care about, or we raised voices and tension interrupted what was meant to be a restful vacation day. Still, at some point we accept that parenting is a complicated life arena that simply can't go well all of the time, or even most of the time. We are parents for life—we can't just toss in the towel and quit—and we bring the same type of understanding to our careers, our education, and other important life areas. We stay the course, take the challenges as they come, learn what works and what doesn't, and move forward. We understand that life's not perfect.

In my coaching around creating lasting changes in healthy behaviors, however, I rarely see people bring this approach to eating and exercise. Instead, we create an idealized goal that aims for an idealized self, especially intertwined with weight pressures and beauty norms and self-worth. We stuff all of this into a motivation bubble so overinflated it can't help but burst upon the tiniest impact with life. We see ourselves as less than perfect in relation to these perfect goals, and as more deserving of our blame when we can't achieve that perfection we're aiming for.

But the truth is, we are complex beings living in a complex world. Healthy eating and physical movement are just two elements of the *whole* of our lives. Think about it—are you primarily a person trying to eat according to a plan or work exercise into your daily routine, or is there more to you than that? The many moving parts in my own life that compete with my own efforts to eat well and stay active include work (and its subparts: researching, speaking, coaching, writing, and consulting), friending, parenting, partnering, daughtering, sistering, grocery shopping, cooking, list making, appointment keeping, dog walking…And on any given day, I need to value some of these more highly than others. An important call from my mom may cut into time allotted for research or I may need to take the dog to the vet when I had planned a walk.

It just depends, right? Life's not perfect. We all know this about our lives, and we move our priorities around without much trouble, while simultaneously stumbling over our artificially inflated eating and exercise bubble. When a point of conflict arises—when our eating plan is challenged by a tempting dish or our bike ride is challenged by a sudden storm—it can feel like a crisis. We *could* follow the same path we take with conflicts to our work or family plans by doing a *part* of our eating or exercise plan, or we could just give up and try again next year. Typically, when facing these ominous conflicts to our ideal eating or exercise plan, we feel overwhelmed and it's all too easy to give up. But it doesn't have to be that way.

FOREVER BLOWING BUBBLES

Just for now, think of all the bits and pieces of your life as bubbles.

We've got a lot of separate bubbles moving around in our daily lives. Work, family, health, finances, and housing are the big ones,

MY DAY

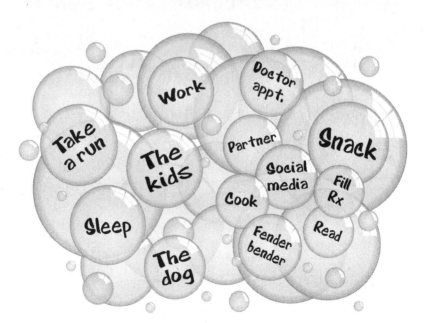

the ones we naturally prioritize. Some are larger, some are smaller. Some rise to the top, some fall to the bottom or cling to the sides. They bump up against one another all the time. Sometimes when they collide, they burst on impact; sometimes one or two bubbles merge, changing direction as they do. These life bubbles are dynamic, changing size and always on the move.

When we embark on a new eating strategy or exercise regimen, to finally be all that we can be, our eating or exercise plan bubble tends to get overinflated, obscuring all of our other life bubbles. Perhaps because it is idealized and it contains our perfect goal, we believe it will never burst. But then life happens. Our eating and exercise bubble bumps up against a higher-priority bubble like work or family and bursts on impact, sending all our plans (and aspirations) right down the drain.

LIFE BURSTS THE MOTIVATION BUBBLE

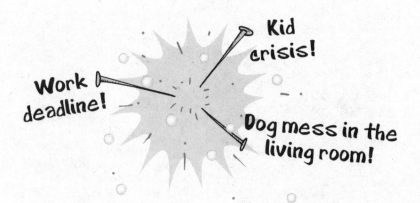

As physiological beings, we have a real need to care for our bodies. Just to stay alive, we need to get enough food, water, and sleep, and to some degree move our bodies. But to do more than *just* survive, we also need to live our lives, fulfilling meaningful life roles—as employees, students, entrepreneurs, clinicians, professionals, creators, coaches, friends, parents, partners, caregivers. At any given time, a different bit of our life suddenly rises to the top of the priority list, needing our attention and our care and, in the process, often creating a very real conflict with our eating or exercise plan.

This point of conflict becomes our *choice point*: the true place of power. What we do here determines not only the fate of our specific eating and exercise plans, but our success in supporting the greater goals they aim to achieve. The Joy Choice, based on the assumption that many of the plans we make *do not work out*, is all about learning to effortlessly and joyfully negotiate those choice points. And a big part of that is having beliefs and strategies that work for rather than against you and all the meaningful things that make up your life.

MEET THE JOY CHOICE

Most often, our strategies to change our eating and exercise behavior begin by following programs, solutions, or rules. Most of them offer us a formula for success, put us on the starting line, and send us off to the eating and exercise races! This standard behavior change formula is a valid and often helpful way to approach changing our behavior. But too often, what happens is that we reach a choice point—Eat the fruit I planned or the donut I want? Go out for my walk or finish that project for work?—and the whole shebang crashes.

Once I started thinking about the fact that it is our *in-the-moment* choices that determine whether we ultimately achieve lasting change, I came to my own choice point in my work: Would I keep doing what I was doing, or would I shift my professional focus to understanding how to resolve the most common conflicts between real life and our intended eating and exercise plans? Not a hard choice. Always seeking to crack the next code, I jumped into this new lane.

Right away, I learned that our general strategies for navigating our eating and exercise choice points determine whether we achieve our greater goals and long-term aspirations. But—and this is very important—the choice point pertains to our exercise and eating *plans*, not to the greater *goals* these plans are in service of achieving. I also began to see that the plans we create for ourselves concern the near-term, what we will do next week, tomorrow, or at dinner tonight. And as we've seen, our intentions and plans bite the dust when stress, anxiety, and too much to do momentarily disrupt our executive functioning, preventing it from keeping us on track with our goals. **So, the solution becomes learning how to successfully navigate these choice points—the never-ending challenges that our specific eating and exercise plans confront—so we can stay on the path, even when there is an unavoidable detour.**

It's not just common sense. Research suggests that our strategies for negotiating unplanned challenges at choice points influence our coping and what transpires.[1] Regardless of what we aspire to achieve through our eating and exercise initiatives, wouldn't it be more strategic for us to learn the tactical beliefs and strategies that can guide us successfully through the rough waters we will inevitably encounter at the choice point?

Our choice points are not only about what we will eat and how we will exercise. We also bring our entire history, beliefs, attitudes, and memories about eating and exercise to *each* and *every* choice point we face, and we do it in the midst of the unpredictable chaos of our daily lives. If that sounds like a lot, that's because it is! But it is also the place of power for achieving lasting change. Which brings us to the Joy Choice, the always-changing compromise that lets you take a moment to play with the possibilities and needs of *this* moment and make the trade-offs that balance those life elements in perfectly *imperfect* ways.

TRADE-OFF THINKING

The opposite of *all-or-nothing* thinking is this: *Something is always better than nothing.* When it comes to achieving lasting changes in eating, exercise, and other self-care behaviors, making strategic trade-offs and compromises in our plans are vital to long-term success.

In a recently published review about trade-offs in choice,[2] the authors explain that most choice problems are resolved by one of two solutions: extreme versus mixed. *Extreme solutions* reflect our old frenemy *all-or-nothing* thinking, making a choice that satisfies a single consideration at the complete expense of another. The most flexible strategy, *mixed solutions*, reflects a compromise that is able to "partially satisfy multiple considerations."

Remember Stephanie's multifamily beach vacation? Following a satisfying dinner, she reached a choice point regarding whether to eat the chocolate cake or not. She only saw an extreme trade-off solution: to join everyone else in eating the cake. This would accommodate them but negate her own need to follow her new eating plan and continue with her otherwise successful changes she had made in her eating. Trapped by Accommodation, Stephanie could only see one extreme trade-off solution, eating the piece of chocolate cake.

How we think about things determines how we see them, experience them, and ultimately determines our future related choices. Had Stephanie framed her choice point differently, she would have seen that other alternatives and possibilities were open to her. She could have decided to eat a smaller slice, or to replace cake with an alternative dessert food that would have felt more aligned with her eating plan. Or she simply could have replaced dessert altogether with a non-food-related celebratory comment or toast to the group, showing she was fully present at this special time. Any of those options, while imperfect, would still have been a double win, permitting Stephanie to honor her valued changes in eating while still joining in on the celebration and honoring the needs of the greater community.

SOME OTHER POSSIBILITIES

Eat a smaller slice

Have an alternative dessert

Non-food celebratory comment

I really like the concept of mixed-solution trade-offs for our eating and exercise choices. Framed this way, we can more clearly see the dynamic context of decision making, and see *choice* and *compromise* rather than only *success* or *failure*. This idea reflects one of the most important overarching assumptions of the Joy Choice solution.

IN THE FRAME

We build our eating and exercise plans and strategies based on the way we frame eating and exercise. I can't stress this point enough: The frame we put around our eating and exercise choices *matters*.

I saw this clearly a few years ago, when my colleagues and I were investigating how women who were regularly active ("high active") framed physical activity as a priority compared to those who were not regularly physically active ("low active").[3] The comments from our focus groups were an eye-opener. The typical comments from low-active women expressed that they framed being active as needing to be perfect, with inflexible standards and all-or-nothing thinking. Referring to exercise, one participant said: "You have to do this at this time, and you have to commit to these hour-long sessions...it's a lot of pressure...I can't commit." Their comments emphasized the kind of thinking that underlies the Perfection trap, so it's not surprising that those who framed exercise in this way also did not participate much in physical activity. They got tired just thinking about it! No wonder they most frequently chose not to do it.

The high-active participants' comments were quite different. They saw physical activity through the frame of flexibility. Some days they were active, and some, they were not. They commented that "it's not the end of the world" if they do not exercise on any given day. As one woman explained, "If we have to spend the long nights [helping] my son on a homework assignment, the workout needs to go on the wayside, so be it.... You have to give and take." These women were flexible with how they framed exercise, and with how they fit exercise into their lives. The result might be less exercise at any given point; but their framing of exercise as needing to *integrate with the other important parts of their lives* kept them on track and active.

This simple reframing easily translates to real-world practice. Sometimes just knowing that you can look at things in a different way can jog you into action. My client Lawrence, for example, was elated when he told me about his success with a recent perfect *imperfect* choice. He had come to coaching feeling like he never had any energy, and his goal was to turn this around. Despite his lifelong dread of exercising, he knew it could help his energy level and was now determined to learn how to become more active in ways that would last. I was impressed with his progress—through the *No Sweat* method, he had quickly learned how to transform exercise from feeling like a chore into feeling like a gift. He liked the activities he was choosing, which also felt gentle on his joints. His favorite was using the elliptical while listening to interesting podcasts. He started out slowly to prevent injury, and after a while found that he was working out for forty-five minutes. After a couple of months, Lawrence told me that he had more energy and confidence, just what he was after. But then he hit a snag.

"I was about to start using the elliptical," he said. "I was dressed and ready to go. Just as I was about to get on the machine, my buddy Tim texted me for help with a programming glitch he'd run into at work. I knew he was under a deadline, and I wanted to help. My old response would have been to drop the exercise altogether, call him back, and then later feel like crap about missing my activity time. But I remembered what you and I had discussed last week and the light went on. Instead of thinking about it as *all*-*or*-*nothing*, I realized that I had some options and could make it fit if I did part of my plan instead of getting stuck in my old way of thinking. Talking things through with Tim as I walked was an option, but I realized doing the elliptical for less time was my preference. I texted him back to call me in twenty-five minutes, which gave me twenty minutes to exercise. It wasn't my ideal, and I didn't have time to shower, but it worked."

This may not sound like a big deal, but this simple success was an epiphany for Lawrence. Seeing his choice points through this new frame opened the floodgates to permit workable alternatives that he would have never before considered worth doing. Hearing about these breakthroughs in my clients' thinking *never* gets old for me.

Quick, look at the following picture. What do you see?

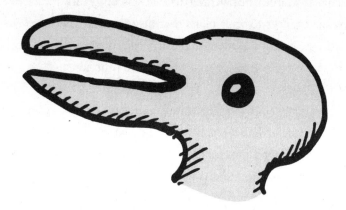

Depending on how you look, you may see either a long-billed bird or a rabbit. Two very different animals! Changing the frame literally determines what we see. Paying attention to how we frame our eating and exercise choices can be a real eye-opener!

Changing the frame at a choice point means that instead of asking ourselves, *Will I do this or not?* we ask, *How can I make this work?* Finding the answer to this new question requires the understanding that a "perfect" choice is rarely feasible; but the perfect *imperfect* option is always available.

There's a reason why Lawrence's dilemma kick-started some problem solving. These seemingly innocuous choice points (such as how to stay on track with your eating plan when you have to go out to lunch with a client) are the type of novel situations that actually trigger our executive functions to come into play.[4] Trust me, this is a team you want on your side.

MEET YOUR EXECUTIVE FUNCTIONING TEAM!

What if you had a management team that was always available to help you think through a new situation or coach you to get past an unanticipated challenge, inhibit unwanted distractions, and motivate you to make the flexible changes to your plans that help you stay the course toward your ultimate eating and exercise goals? Well, congratulations. You do!

These are your three primary executive functions:

+ *Working memory* is the small and ever-changing amount of information that we can hold and work with in our mind at one time, helping us focus our attention so we compare options, make trade-offs, and enact our new plans.
+ *Flexible thinking* reflects our ability to switch gears, tasks, or tactics in the moment so that we can successfully meet challenges and stay the path.
+ *Inhibition* helps us resist acting on impulse, setting the stage to make a choice more aligned with our plans and goals.

Each of these three executive functions is powerful in its own right, but they form a set of abilities that we might think of as our *executive functioning team*.

MY EXECUTIVE FUNCTIONING TEAM

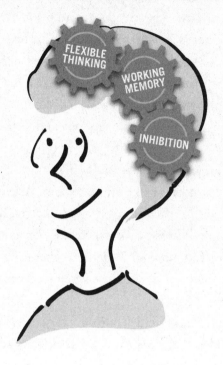

Associated with neural activity in the areas of our prefrontal cortex, this set of higher-level cognitive capacities and skills enable us humans to deliberate, focus our attention, hold and work with information that is temporarily stored in our short-term working memory, and successfully pursue our long-term goals.[5] These wonderful mental abilities evolved to help us deal with novel challenges, like unexpected conflicts.[6] When engaged and working together, this underlying brain-based mechanism helps you make lasting changes in eating and exercise. Your executive functions help you interact with Perfection in productive ways and enable you to override decision traps like Rebellion or Accommodation so you can activate flexible problem solving to resolve any competing needs, just as Lawrence did.

As we've seen, conflict actually invokes executive functioning to help us focus our attention and assess and prioritize our numerous competing daily needs *in the moment.* Unlike an automatic habit, this is a *conscious* process that enables and requires our awareness and attention.[7] When we need them, our executive functions mobilize our thinking, inhibiting our impulse to self-sabotage, redirecting our attention to consider a few better options and decisively choose the best one.

At this point, you may be feeling like Tom, who said he'd always struggled with learning; or like my new client, Arielle, a student and young mother with a part-time job, who told me flat out that her life was "too complicated" to learn something as complex sounding as executive functioning. Whether genetically or circumstantially, we differ in our innate abilities when it comes to our executive functioning.

I'll tell you what I told Tom and Arielle: No hard labor is required here! In fact, the opposite. These abilities are already part of our brain's operating system—not something we need to work hard to "learn," as much as something we can *support* through strategies like joy, play, and strategic easy-to-remember acronyms (you'll learn these in the next chapter!). Combined, these strategies help us simplify how we think about our options, and then we just let them do their thing. As with so many important parts of our lives, we can change our frame guided by new, scientifically supported (and playful) ways of thinking to get better results.

The Joy Choice solution was explicitly designed to support these three primary executive functions—working memory, flexible thinking, and inhibition—in service of successfully navigating your eating and exercise choice points. The next three chapters dive into each function and the new ways of thinking you can use to support it. Then, in the last two chapters, you'll see how you can put these ideas to work in your own life using the Joy Choice decision tool POP!, and we'll wrap things up by coming full circle in "Learning Lasting Change." By the end, you'll have learned very positive ideas and specific science-based tactics that will set you up to achieve the lasting changes with eating and exercise you've always been after.

⤜nine⤛

SIMPLIFY: SUPPORTING WORKING MEMORY

"I'M STRESSED AND OUT OF CONTROL OF MY EATING, AND MOST DAYS, IT'S impossible for me to find time for even a short walk," my client Patty said at our first meeting. When I asked her what she thought was getting in her way, she gave me a familiar—and wildly understated—explanation that, on the surface, had nothing to do with eating or exercise. "I have three young kids," she said. "And I know that if I don't write something on my to-do list, I'll forget, but I don't even have time to do that!"

As she shared more details, I learned that her mind was constantly overwhelmed by the truckload of things she needed to think about and keep track of—including her own personal and professional needs, her three children's needs, her husband's needs, and their household needs (including pets). Add to that, she had recently become more and more worried about and distracted by her parents' health concerns, and her anxiety about them had left her feeling out of control.

"My mind feels like a tornado of to-dos," she said. "I can't seem to ever accomplish anything." She explained that as she tries to finish one single, little to-do (putting vegetables on the shopping list), she suddenly realizes that she forgot to leave water out for the dog. This new to-do pushes her grocery list to-do out of her mind. But it doesn't stop there. The dog to-do gets pushed out by the next one (making sure all three kids had their homework), and then the next one (calling the plumber to fix the leaky faucet), and on and on and on! This is both stressful and frustrating, and it happens almost every day. Not surprisingly, it's a disaster for her new healthy eating plans. All this chaos easily crashes her working memory capacity, preventing Patty from inhibiting her impulse to open the cupboard and reach for a candy bar instead of eating her planned meal.

HOW WORKING MEMORY WORKS

Our working memory is meant for *working*: Temporarily holding and processing bits of information that we can use in the moment. It's like a container for that information, but its storage capacity is small.[1] As soon as a new thought pops into our mind, it easily shoves out the other thought that we had just been thinking. Annoying, yes; but that's the way it works. Most of us can only hold a couple of thoughts in our mind at the same time,[2] far short of the true complexity that we have to deal with in our daily lives.

But working memory isn't just the container of fleeting thoughts and memories. It's also the gatekeeper of our long-term memory. Its capacity at a given time influences our ability to focus, manage, and use key information.[3] Clearly, when our mind is bouncing frantically between all of our many to-dos, as Patty's is, our scattered attention can't escape being sucked right into the swirling vortex of that tornado.

TORNADO OF TO-DOS

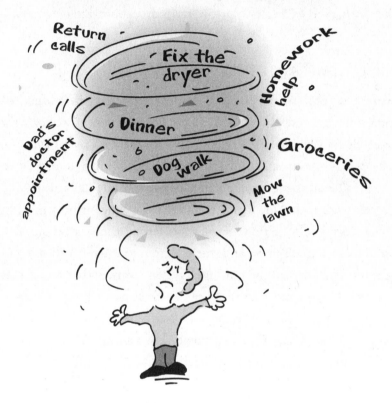

Whether or not you have three children, a partner, and a dog added to your busy life equation, daily life can be and often is chaotic. When we are stressed, anxious, and have a lot of things on our mind, our working memory easily gets blown to smithereens. ADHD (attention deficit/hyperactivity disorder) and executive functioning expert Joel Nigg, PhD, puts it succinctly: "When a worry or 'to-do' enters your mind, something else has to go. It's as if twenty people are talking to you, but ten of them are in your own head."[4] Yikes.

It can feel impossible to stay on task, whether for eating, exercise, or some other important life area, especially when we're in the middle of the information overload. But as the title of this chapter suggests, we can use some simple strategies to organize the mess and simplify the chaos. And we begin where we started, with working memory.

WHY I LOVE WORKING MEMORY

Here's my confession: When I began to explore executive functioning to develop tools for my coaching clients, I avoided reading the research on working memory because it just seemed *dull*: I thought, what's sexy about something I (then!) had (wrongly!) pegged as merely a small mental container? But my attitude has turned 180 degrees since then. Now I understand that working memory isn't just about storing information for the short term.[5] It influences our ability to focus our attention and shield it from interference, helping us suppress our worries[6] and cravings.[7] When I learned that we actually need working memory to simplify our decision making by *keeping out distractions so that our eating and exercise plans stay active, in the forefront of our minds* at a choice point,[8] I was a convert.

So, how can we help? Regular physical activity and exercise are considered to be among the very best things we can do throughout our lives to benefit our executive functioning, and working memory tasks in particular[9]—including focusing, organizing, and flexibly responding to situations as needed.[10] These effects are so potent that physical activity is considered one of the very best ways to treat conditions like ADHD.[11] These exercise-induced cognitive benefits not only help kids learn and perform better in school, and help adults stave off devastating illnesses like Alzheimer's; the research suggests that regular physical activity helps *all of us* think better.[12]

Time-out. I know that you might be reading this book because you are challenged to get the regular type of physical activity you need to achieve these benefits. Fear not! We're on our way in this chapter to the fun and easy-to-remember POP! decision tool (hint: POP = Pause, Open up your options and play, and Pick the Joy Choice), which will help you do just that. Okay, back to our tale.

Working memory really got my attention and respect the moment that I understood its central role in supporting our other executive functions, such as our ability to inhibit self-sabotaging impulses and to think flexibly when problem solving. These abilities are critical to helping us sustain healthy eating and exercise alike. To devise any plan of action or make a choice, we need to be able to keep the relevant information in our working memory. For example, if I start to walk my dog, can't recall where I put the leash, and forget my house key, I'm in big trouble.

Working memory has been called "the most important among the various executive functions";[13] and in his best-selling book *SPARK: The Revolutionary New Science of Exercise and the Brain*, neuropsychiatrist John Ratey calls working memory the *backbone* of the executive functions.[14] So, I admit it: I got working memory *very* wrong. Working memory is *awesome*.

CAN APPS BOOST OUR WORKING MEMORY?

So, supporting working memory is a great idea. Given its critical role in making healthy exercise and eating choices, it's no wonder that a whole multibillion-dollar industry and area of research is centrally focused on boosting its capacity. I agree that it would be wonderful if all we had to do was buy an app or do some memory training to accomplish this feat. Unfortunately, it doesn't work that way.

Perhaps the best known of the "brain games" companies is Lumosity, which aims to train everything from speed and flexibility to mindfulness and math—and working memory. Lumosity touts published research on its website as evidence of its program's effectiveness,[15] and at first glance, the results are impressive. It had some short-term success[16] (as studies in academic settings that are not selling a product like Lumosity often find too). Despite small short-term gains from these types of trainings, research shows no evidence that these effects persist over time.[17] The training gains have trouble surviving real-world tasks and problem solving. Even working memory trainings that are gamified (designed to be fun)[18] or designed specifically to help people change their eating and manage health conditions like type 2 diabetes similarly show disappointing results: little or no training effects, no effects beyond those experienced in the control condition, or short-term gains that are lost in the long term.[19]

All of this research and innovation has been premised on a very specific question: Can we design games and tasks in the lab that can boost working memory so we'll eat in better ways at home? But it might be that we've been asking the wrong question when it comes to supporting our working memory capacity. I think the real question we need to ask is this: *When we are facing a challenging food or exercise choice point*, what could best help us support our working memory *in that moment* so we make the choice we'll be happiest with? This question takes us out of the lab and in a completely new direction: how people actually learn to perform tasks in the wilderness of real life.

Successfully sustaining our changes in eating and exercise behaviors over time is the *evidence* that we have learned how to make the consistent eating and exercise decisions that underlie sustainability. The key word here is *learning*: If we automatically knew how to do it, there would have been no need for me to write this book!

REAL-WORLD KNOWLEDGE

Would you rather take a cross-country flight with a pilot who's had one hundred hours of simulation training, perfect scores on his written tests, but only a few hours of real flight time, or with an experienced pilot who was a mediocre student but left the classroom long ago and has safely flown thousands of miles in a variety of weather conditions? No contest, right? The veteran pilot who has learned the ins and outs of flying in a variety of real-world contexts holds what Julie Dirksen, author of *Design for How People Learn*,[20] calls *real* knowledge: knowledge that we can retrieve and use right when we need it.

I love coaching people on how to make sustainable changes in lifestyle behaviors, but the first time I was asked to teach others how to do what I do, I panicked. I had no idea how I did it; I just did it! Maybe you've found yourself in the same predicament. When we know how to do something really well, we are considered to be *unconsciously competent*. We can do it, no problem, but since we don't have a *conscious awareness* about how we do it so well, we can't very well teach others how to do it.

Thankfully, the learning and development industry is centrally focused on the "how-tos" of training professionals like me to become consciously competent so I can teach others what I know. Since that time, I have been an eager student of this knowledge base. One of my core takeaways from this process takes us directly back to working memory.[21]

Memory is powerful when it comes to influencing our exercise and eating-related choices. Full, rich memories, like that tempting memory of eating a chocolate croissant with our friends, are encoded into our seemingly infinite long-term memory where they are grouped with similar memories. With the right cue—in this case, seeing the croissant—the memory of that satisfying moment flows into our working memory.

Of course, it's not all pastries in there! Our love and concern for our families, our regard for our work, and our valued fitness plans and eating goals are in there, and can also be cued to show up in our transitory working memory. Once there, they can remind us of what we care about achieving and help us make a reasoned choice.

The great news is that we can support our beleaguered working memory by using science-based strategies to help us retrieve these self-care-facilitating long-term memories. *Retrieval*, the technical word for recalling information stored in long-term memory, is the necessary *first* step that allows us to manipulate, combine, and innovate with the information we hold in working memory. But successful retrieval necessitates that we *first* successfully store, or encode, this information into our long-term memory so it's ready to pull out when needed.[22]

GETTING INTO LONG-TERM MEMORY

The strategic info we want to store in long-term memory has to first be relevant enough to pass through the gate of working memory. The memories that make it into storage are, well, memorable. Julie Dirksen explains: "Some of the jump to long-term memory is utility— should I hang on to this because I'll use it in the future? Some of it is novelty—if it was really unusual, it will stick. Some of it is familiarity or relevance—I've seen this a lot before."[23]

The useful memories are those you use over and over again, such as your address or your Social Security number, or other familiar things (your pet's name, your favorite songs as a young teen). Some "unusual" memories that make it in contain information that is very emotional, including happy memories (seeing your newborn for the first time, swimming a mile of laps in the pool, a wonderful meal you ate on vacation) and sad or painful ones (a cutting remark that you heard as a child, where you were when you heard about a tragedy). Or—and this is the one we want to play with here—it gets into long-term memory simply because it is *relevant and meaningful to our daily life and the things we value.*

This last reason is the most important for our purposes in picking the Joy Choice: If the information we need to make our in-the-moment eating and exercise choices is sufficiently relevant, it can go from our working memory into our long-term memory. You can do this by strategically "packaging" the information in ways that make it easier to encode it. And when we visualize information, literally picturing it via images in our mind, it can help us remember a lot.[24] (For example, you might visualize placing each item on your grocery shopping list in a different place in your house to help you recall the list when you're at the store.) But a simple and popular memory strategy (*mnemonic*) is one you are likely already familiar with: acronyms.

An *acronym* is a word formed by using the first letter of each word that you want to combine in a way that is meaningful and easy to remember. Acronyms are so helpful, and actually fun. You may be familiar with the BRAT diet—eating bananas, rice, applesauce, and toast to soothe an upset stomach. (Thankfully, there is no image for this one!) Or if you ever studied music as a child, you may have remembered the treble clef (EGBDF) as the sentence "Every good boy deserves fruit."

AVOIDING YOUR TRAPS

We've already made the four classic decision disruptors easy to remember by giving them memorable names (Temptation, Rebellion, Accommodation, and Perfection) whose first letters *also* create the acronym TRAP to remind us of the automatic and unexpected ways they interfere. With this acronym in place, we can bring our TRAPs to awareness and work with them much more productively.

As I was thinking about mnemonics, I came across research that found when children "label" a phenomenon in a meaningful way it helps their executive functioning, including encouraging flexible thinking and focusing attention. This makes a lot of sense. Labeling affords us a sort of cognitive control over our experience,[25] helping us become *experts* on our own experience and allowing us to think about and work with it in productive ways. When we have a label for something, regardless of our age, it puts a name on our experience, representing it in a meaningful way. This makes it easier to grasp, recall, and work with in our mind—the very thing that benefits our working memory capacity at the choice point.

Beyond these benefits, putting the name TRAP on our decision-disrupting beliefs and memories immediately puts us into the observer role. This moves us smoothly from reactive to reflective and allows us to retake the reins of our experience. Author Dan Siegel, clinical professor of psychiatry at the UCLA School of Medicine and executive director of the Mindsight Institute, describes this benefit succinctly: "name it to tame it." Simply naming the TRAPs we encounter at an eating and exercise choice point puts some distance between us and them and gives us the space we need to figure out our next strategic steps. So, let's get to that!

POP! YOUR PLAN: INTRODUCING THE JOY CHOICE DECISION TOOL

Ultimately, no matter how great our plan, sooner or later it is going to bump up against a conflict. This conflict creates the choice point: We can't do what we planned, so what are we going to do now? Choice points are all about logistics—managing our plans and resources. Our old go-to, all-or-nothing thinking, can only result in "nothing" because "all" is no longer possible. So, when we arrive at a choice point, the options are "nothing" or "something else." Choosing "something else" means reframing the moment as a true choice point so we can create a workaround with the resources currently at our disposal.

Wouldn't it be great if we had an easy way to navigate these logistics and our choice points? Well, we do, and it's called POP!—the Joy Choice decision tool. Just like TRAP, the POP! acronym is easy to remember and use when we need it. In Chapter 12, we'll dive deeper into the details of how POP! embodies the three executive functioning strategies and how you can use it in your own life; but for now, you'll see how it guides us step by step to picking the Joy Choice through Lois's story:

⇒POP!⇐ LOIS LEANS INTO POP!

Let's start by looking at the plan that Lois made for exercising. She had an aboveground pool in her backyard. During our session, she had created her plan for the coming week: four days of walking in the pool for thirty minutes while listening to music she liked to dance to. She planned to do this at around five in the afternoon as a way to transition from work to family life. It was Monday, her first day, and she was excited to start her new exercise plan using these new ideas.

After work, she changed into her bathing suit and brought her portable speakers outside. Her young son, Alex, was being watched by her visiting in-laws, so that life area was being taken care of. But just as she stepped into the pool, she heard Alex bawling from the window—he had discovered that his mom was about to enter his favorite place, the pool, without him.

Lois stopped in her tracks, flooded with guilt and ready to go back inside and comfort Alex. At the same moment, she also recalled the phrase we'd talked about memorizing at our last coaching session—**"Conflict = Choice Point"**—and the accompanying image automatically appeared in her head, getting her attention fast!

LIFE IS HAPPENING, CONFLICTS ARISE...
It's a choice point!

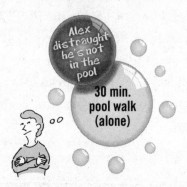

Without a mental structure for easily handling challenges to our plan, it's easy to lose focus by the swirl of disappointment, worry about the conflict, and the deeper TRAPs we could fall into. The POP! process avoids all of that and puts us back in control immediately: All we have to do is POP! our plan. And that's just what Lois did.

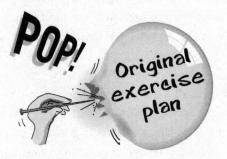

Pause
Open up your options and play
Pick the Joy Choice

POP! is not just an acronym, it's also the metaphorical action that pops our plan bubble, freeing us up to figure out what else we can do. As a working memory support, POP! is depicted with graphics, and it has three simple, easy-to-remember steps (listed in our POP! graphic).

1. Pause

PAUSE

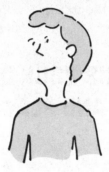

The Pause might seem simplistic and not worth doing. But it is actually the opposite! The incredible value of pausing can't be overstated. It is the mechanism that creates the space we need to most effectively improvise at choice points. Lois paused, took a slow breath, and let it out. This gave her the space to inhibit her usual Accommodation disruptor from pulling her focus elsewhere, and she immediately felt that her mind was back in her body rather than upstairs with Alex.

Then, she said to herself, "Lois, you can do this. It doesn't have to be perfect." Getting some distance helps us understand that while we *have* these feelings, thoughts, and experiences, we *are not* our feelings or our experiences. We can then step back, observe, and choose with intention.

Lois noticed that she felt some guilt about having been away from Alex all day and then going to the pool instead of spending time with him. But within the space created by the Pause she softly said, "Accommodation, I see you. But I'm moving on."

And with that, she moved on to the next step.

2. **O**pen up your options and play

To identify what else might work, we need to open our options by identifying alternative possibilities and playing with them. Lois recognized it was the end of the day, and that it would be hard to find another time she could fit in a different physical activity. But she and I had already discussed how easy it was to think outside of the box when we POP! our plan. She thought

OPEN UP YOUR OPTIONS AND PLAY

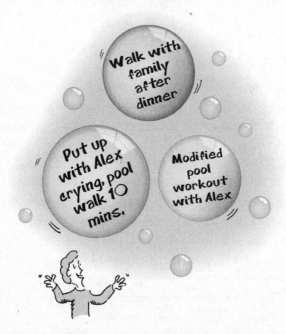

Walk with family after dinner

Put up with Alex crying, pool walk 10 mins.

Modified pool workout with Alex

about her options. She could try to bear her son's screaming and do her pool walk for just ten minutes, but that felt completely joyless. Another option would be to bring Alex into the pool with her, changing the activity. Or she realized she could invite her full extended family to take a walk after dinner.

She thought about the logistics as she played with these possibilities to figure out which one was best that day.

3. Pick the Joy Choice

Lois realized that the Joy Choice would be to do her pool workout with Alex. That way, she got some fun exercise, and she also helped meet her son's needs.

Pick the Joy Choice

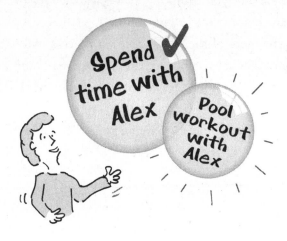

Once she realized that this was her perfect *imperfect* option *for today*, she called up to her in-laws to bring Alex down to the pool, dressed for swimming, and got five minutes to herself before they came down.

When Lois told me about this at her next session, I asked her what she had taken into account in picking that Joy Choice. She said that she had recognized that she had been away at work the full day, away from Alex, and that was the key input she used to make her Joy Choice calculation. "Michelle, to tell you the truth, when I think about it now, it really wasn't much of a trade-off. Sure, I didn't get the harder, dance-infused water-walking workout I had planned. But it felt good to realize that I could change up a couple of things and meet *both* of these needs."

POP! quickly liberates us from what no longer works and opens us up to a myriad of possibilities. You can use POP! with any program or plan, anywhere and anytime because it's a tool to cut through the noise and guide your thinking, strategically helping you navigate through the choice point to picking the Joy Choice. And the more you do it, the more of the POP! decision process will become successfully encoded into your long-term memory, ready and waiting for you when it's needed. Plus, let's admit it, popping bubbles is just fun anyway!

And fun is exactly what we are using to fuel the Joy Choice. So, let's move on to Play, the next chapter!

ten

PLAY: SUPPORTING FLEXIBLE THINKING

A FEW WEEKS AGO, I SPONTANEOUSLY STOPPED BY MY FRIEND CHERI'S house and invited her to join me on a walk. She opened the door barefoot, dressed in her yoga clothes and holding her mat under her arm. I wasn't surprised when she regretfully declined my invitation, explaining that she was about to start her daily yoga routine.

But as I turned and started down the sidewalk to continue on my own, she suddenly yelled after me, "Wait! I'm coming with you! I just have to put on my trainers."

I was happy, but surprised. "I thought you couldn't walk today because you were doing yoga?"

Cheri laughed. "I reevaluated. Today, spending time with you will be my yoga."

Because Cheri was open to being flexible about her plans, she was able to let go of her specific yoga plan and play with some other possibilities—like spending time with a friend (me!), going for a relaxing walk, having an engaging conversation—and she quickly

chose to trade her yoga activity with another activity that was consistent with her goal to be physically active but also brought her a
fuller joy *in that moment.*

And this is a key component of the Joy Choice: *The value of any
choice always depends on the context of the other possibilities.*[1] Cheri would
have been just fine following through with her planned yoga, but she
explained her choice this way: "Michelle, I love yoga—I feel clearer
and calmer from it. But once walking with you became a possibility,
I realized that I would not only get similar mind-body benefits, but
it would be fun, too. We always laugh a lot when we're together." She
was able to recognize this because her goal was *not* to do yoga every
day at a particular time, but to stay physically active more generally.
She let herself play with the possible alternatives to her scheduled
plan when they arose, and went with the one that brought her the
most joy that day. Her choice not only inserted variety into her workouts, something that increases intrinsic motivation[2] (a key predictor
of long-term participation), but possibly even boosted her self-care
quotient. But I am clearly biased on that matter!

Similar principles apply across all of our opportunities to choose,
whether they are as straightforward as Cheri's or more fraught with
challenges: When we liberate ourselves from rigid all-or-nothing
thinking and start to believe that in most cases, doing something
is better than doing nothing, we free ourselves to enter into a more
colorful and expansive world of new possibilities we can play with.

PLAY—IT'S NOT JUST FOR KIDS

Play is not a concept we generally associate with eating plans and
exercise regimens, but it's a fundamental premise of the Joy Choice.
Playing is the opposite of "shoulding" and all-or-nothing thinking.
There are a lot of science-based reasons to allow more playtime into

our lives, but perhaps the number one reason we want to play is because it's *fun*.

Play is universal. It occurs in birds and across higher-functioning animals, even across the life stages for high-functioning mammals, like us.[3] Play can be enjoyable *and* promote skill building *at the same time*. Free play is "fun, voluntary, challenging, relaxed, carefree, spontaneous, pleasurable, flexible, and characterized by intrinsic motivation. Play is the essence of being human."[4] It engages us and helps us focus our attention.

Please note: When we talk about Play as basic to the Joy Choice, we are most definitely *not* talking about a game you can win or lose. We're talking about the joy of free play, which allows us to explore new options, to try on new ideas to see how they fit, to learn what we like and don't like, and what we'd like to try again. When it comes to the Joy Choice, play is a no-fail activity. We can't hold back the ever-shifting nature of daily demands and needs that create unexpected conflicts. But rather than toss in the towel at our choice points, we can choose to play with our possibilities and keep making strides toward the consistency that underlies lasting change.

When for so long the automatic, rote, and perfect have ruled behavior change and deviation from the plan has equaled failure, this idea might sound radical. I get this. But hear me out.

IT'S A BIRD, IT'S A PLANE…IT'S FLEXIBLE THINKING TO THE RESCUE!

Flexibility is considered *the* cognitive style needed for societies to flourish, and is a prerequisite for successful innovation across life areas within our modern world.[5] Flexible thinking is associated with a better quality of life and well-being, and is considered to be a fundamental aspect of health. It cultivates psychological resilience to negative life events, including better coping and emotion regulation within work, relationships, and leisure.[6]

I'm banging the flexibility drum so loudly for a good reason. We've been told over and over again, across decades, to *stick to the plan no matter what*. This idea is so deeply embedded in our psyches that inevitably these inflexible plans get blown to smithereens, leaving us picking up the pieces, once again despondent and pessimistic about ever becoming successful. But flexible thinking is our true superpower when it comes to successfully navigating choice points and making consistent decisions. Let's talk about that.

By *consistent* I don't mean making the same choices all of the time. I mean making the decisions and choices that support and are in harmony with our long-term goals, core values, and identity, just like we do for most of our other life areas. For example, Cheri demonstrated flexibility when she was willing to change up her routine that day. And she demonstrated consistency when she realized that walking, like yoga, supported her goal of staying active on most days, and it also resonated with her core values of friendship and connection. Just as several different paths may all take you to the same lake on any given day, consistent choices by their very nature will vary from day to day. But *they* are what bring us to lasting change.

PLAYING WITH THE POSSIBILITIES

I'm not the first person to assert the benefits of playing with the possibilities; this phrase is in the air. In the Joy Choice, playing with the options at our eating and exercise choice points is designed to be a fun opportunity rather than a grim obligation. In fact, a playful, open attitude is *precisely* the mindset we need to stay the course over the long term. And flexible thinking is what makes that happen.

Flexible thinking (also called cognitive flexibility, or set shifting) is the executive function underlying our ability to pivot and switch tasks or strategies in the moment.[7] This ability to be nimble to meet the changes in our day enables us to stay on track by rethinking a thwarted plan, devising an alternative strategy, or even just disengaging if a bad night's sleep makes taking a break from exercise the best strategy *today*.

Flexible thinking drives creativity and resilience in the face of challenges and unexpected sudden change. As we've seen, studies generally find that when it comes to eating and exercise, being overly restrictive often backfires, throwing us headlong into Temptation or Rebellion. However, flexible thinking enables us to better manage our food consumption and physical activity.[8]

Flexible thinking is recognized as a core health-related resource. It is considered essential for preventing eating disorders in adolescents[9] and also effectively managing arthritis in older populations.[10] In fact, striving toward *any* plan or goal in a flexible way is considered paramount to continued engagement and long-term behavioral pursuit,[11] not only in lifestyle behaviors but across many parts of life. This idea might seem counterintuitive given that the old behavior change story has taught us success comes from the opposite of flexibility, but stay with me.

The power of flexible thinking to help us effectively respond to challenges works in a couple of different ways. One way is that flexible thinking allows us to continue to pursue our lifestyle goals by picking a more effective eating strategy *when the one we had originally planned turns out to be unworkable in real time*. While this idea might sound heretical to health promoters, and to everything society has taught us, research suggests that such flexible reprieves are beneficial.[12]

The evidence that flexible thinking is a key player in maintaining change is mounting. When it comes to using a flexible, permissive eating strategy, it is called "flexible restraint."[13] For example, you might decide to build in a regular reprieve by eating according to plan to the best of your ability during the week, but adding more flexibility to enjoy foods that are not on it over the weekend. Many people find this idea counterintuitive or even a cop-out, yet recent research suggests this is an adaptive strategy.[14]

The other way we win with flexible thinking is that it enables us to make *consistent* choices. One study reported that having greater flexible thinking not only predicted *more* physical activity, but that flexible thinking worked *through people substituting and changing their physical activities*, resulting in more physical activity.[15] That's exactly what Cheri did.

When I share stories like Cheri's about the power of flexible thinking, and actually advocate for *not* following "the plan" when it bumps up against life, people often question her choice. They sometimes even express concern over the long-term impact of letting herself spontaneously change up her exercise plan on a whim. They worry that such flexibility will turn into an automatic and permanent "pass" from doing yoga, or any exercise, for that matter. This is a logical outcome to worry about, and quite common based on their own personal experiences. *This is not what we are talking about here!* The Joy Choice is a mindset refresh that swings you out of "should" jail and into a place where understanding that choosing what feels good—and is also consistent with your goals— is actually what keeps you on track with long-term change.

PRESCRIPTION CONSTRICTION

Sometimes when I'm training clinicians how to teach their patients to play with the possibilities, these professionals express concern about enabling people to do less than the *ideal*. Once during a clinician training, one of my learners abruptly stood up to challenge me. She was upset about my contention that she should give her patients permission to not follow her exercise *prescription* to a T. She asked, "How can you say that it's okay for my patients to walk at a leisurely pace? They won't get the cardiovascular benefits they need to control their illnesses." I paused. I could tell she was angry, and I knew that how I responded would either get the training back on track or send it spiraling out of control. I decided to get right to the point: "How's that working for you?" I asked with a smile. She sat right down.

I've already noted that this book does not offer medical advice, and any choices you might make regarding any health- or illness-related conditions should be discussed with your clinician. There *are* real medical situations in which the prescribed treatment *must* be followed or dire consequences can result. But we still need to understand the ways in which blanket prescriptions from clinicians for changes in lifestyle behaviors like eating and exercise can turn into all-or-nothing thinking for patients for whom the Perfection trap is an old acquaintance.

Medical prescriptions, by their very nature, need to be specific. But when it comes to eating and exercise, for so many of us, life is too complex and chaotic to be able to hit that prescribed mark every time. We complex human beings do not live our lives in a perfectly controlled laboratory, and so what might be "ideal" for better health might not be realistic for patients to regularly achieve. This "prescription dynamic" does not only empower Perfection. It also can create an interpersonal dynamic between clinicians and their patients whereby patients feel like failures, experiencing embarrassment, shame, and anger. And clinicians can experience disappointment in their patients, and even in themselves and their counseling abilities. These experiences not only create a lose-lose outcome, they are not health promoting either. Some of my clients confide that they even skip clinician visits to avoid having these experiences.

This dynamic trickles down through technology, too. Sometimes when I'm consulting on digital behavior change products, I initially discover that rigid thinking has been inadvertently designed right into the user experience. This happens a lot simply because it reflects the traditional rules of behavior change we've learned and internalized so deeply that we often don't realize that we're still thinking this way. Fortunately, modifying an algorithm to cultivate a flexible approach is easy to do.

The irony is clear. Exercise or eating changes are often prescribed in specific doses by health providers, lifestyle coaches, personal trainers, apps, or even an employer to achieve important outcomes like preventing disease or managing an illness. But whatever the motivation, Perfection, by its very nature, is always going to be a trap. So, our task at choice points is to recognize it by its name, give it a shout-out, and kindly send it on its way. Let's see how things play out with Tom's trade-off:

POP! TOM'S POP! TRADE-OFF

> **By the time he was at a party celebrating his nephew's** high school graduation, my client Tom had already had a lot of practice with POP! He arrived at the party with his eating plan in the forefront of his mind. As soon as he surveyed the various food options spread out across the table, he saw that nothing on his plan was on it. Without hesitation, Tom automatically recognized this was a choice point!
>
> ### LIFE IS HAPPENING, CONFLICTS ARISE...
> ### It's a choice point!

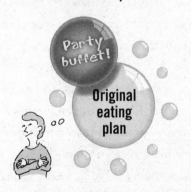

Now that he was at the party and enjoying himself with his family and friends, it occurred to him that part of that experience included eating something special from the buffet that wouldn't be *too* far off from his eating plan, and he knew what to do next—POP! his plan.

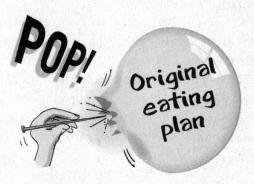

Pause
Open up your options and play
Pick the Joy Choice

1. Pause

PAUSE

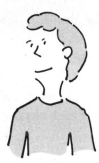

Tom *Paused* before deciding what to do next. Usually, he'd take this time to see if he was about to step into any of his usual TRAPs. But he knew he'd already outsmarted Rebellion by giving himself permission to enjoy something off his plan. However, he did see Temptation up ahead as he recalled memories of past indulgences and started craving them.

Tom remembered the science we'd discussed suggesting that when we mindfully "load up" our working memory with experiences and "occupy it" by visualizing specific things, we can reduce our cravings.[16] And that's what he did. Tom intentionally visualized the POP! sequence of graphics and later told me he had fewer cravings than usual from seeing an enticing food spread like this. Gathering his attention, Tom focused on the next step.

2. Open up your options and play

When we had originally talked about using POP! on the spot as a choice-making tool, Tom told me he was worried that he would have trouble thinking of alternatives in the stress of a foiled plan. But I assured him that the whole purpose of POP! is to help people cut through the noise and the distractions and identify new options through very concrete tactics.

We can best open our options and play with the possibilities when we consider the logistics—or planning aspects—of devising a plan B. Questions to experiment with include:

What else could we do? (What other options exist in that moment or that day for alternative food choices or physical activities?)

When could we implement a part or all of the original plan, if it can't work now?

How much time of an activity or quantity of food could we change to create an acceptable compromise? (What could we change regarding the amount of time we'd originally planned to exercise? Or what's an amount of an "alternative" food choice that is a perfect *imperfect* option and acceptable?)

The goal is *not* to go through each of these questions; they are just there as an aid if you need help identifying other possible options and alternatives.

Here's how Tom thought about some other options and possibilities he could play with at the party and later in the day.

When? He needs something to eat now, at the party. His goal is to do something reasonable instead of going wild.

What else? At first glance, the possible options at the buffet appeared to be deal-breakers—pies, coleslaw, burgers, brownies, potato chips, and roasted potatoes smelling and looking delicious and surrounded by add-ins like butter, cheese,

Open up your options AND PLAY

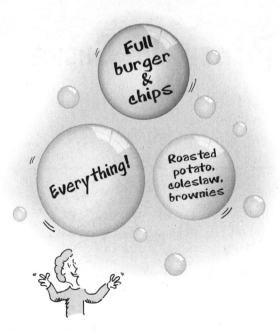

Full burger & chips

Everything!

Roasted potato, coleslaw, brownies

sour cream, and bacon. But Tom had already replaced his old all-or-nothing thinking with the Joy Choice mindset, which gave him permission to find the perfect *imperfect* workable alternative. He saw several options immediately.

How much? *Eating everything* on the table was a possible option, or just leaving hungry and depressed. But having learned how to retake the reins from Temptation, Rebellion, and Perfection, Tom was no longer under their power. Liberated from those old TRAPs, he opened up his options and played with the possibilities that existed at this event and for that day.

3. Pick the Joy Choice

After evaluating the various possibilities, he quickly determined which one he really wanted. He wanted to try a couple of the delicious-looking options but compromised with the *how much*. He chose to eat *half* of a burger and *half* of the roasted potato, sprinkling on a small spoonful of cheese for flavor.

Pick the Joy Choice

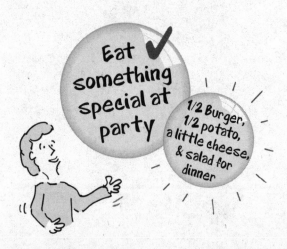

Grounded in the knowledge that he was in charge, no longer following rules he needed to rebel against, and respecting his self-determined eating goals, Tom effortlessly picked this Joy Choice. He knew it wasn't taking him too far off (his) course, and also decided that he'd have a light salad for dinner as part of his choice.

Tom chose the perfect *imperfect* option (for him, at that moment) through flexible thinking and play. His trade-off delivered satisfaction from eating something celebratory at the party, yet still feeling like he respected his general eating plan. His Joy Choice tasted great and he felt proud about how he had arrived at it. This choice and these positive experiences and pride from successfully using the POP! process accompanied him back home with his family, and created new positive memories he could call on at the next choice point.

※ ※ ※

The ownership element here can't be underestimated. You are creating your own eating and exercise story now, and you are *curious* about what else might be possible at this point, what works and what doesn't, what feels right. Your choice isn't about what you *should* do, or following the plan to a T. It's simply one choice out of many that you'll make that week. When we take off the pressure of having to do things "the right way" and become more comfortable with being flexible, we often ultimately achieve more—even if we do that by doing less at a particular choice point than we'd planned.

One of the most important benefits of this type of trade-off thinking is that it inherently implies "choice," and offers the opportunity to create success when two life area needs are on a collision course (like Tom's eating plan *and* his desire to join in the celebratory meal with his community). The Joy Choice lets us take care of our full lives, our individual self, *and* the other parts (friends, family) that make life meaningful. Rather than running headlong into our target without considering other options, trade-off thinking gives us permission to creatively play with what is actually possible in *this* moment. We get to POP! our plan, play, and land on our feet.

This success, in turn, doesn't just increase our confidence in our ability to effectively navigate challenges, it opens us up to get curious, which unlocks the door to a world of options and opportunities we never knew existed. Curiosity—about playing, our likes and dislikes, our choices, and our world—helps drive the Joy Choice. Curiosity did *not* kill the cat, but it may have enabled her to identify the easiest way to get her food and affection needs met. For us humans, curiosity is considered a positive emotion, and a motivating force, and an ingredient to well-being.[17] It harnesses our intrinsic motivation,[18] propelling us to explore the ins and outs of the problem we want to solve, finding new information and drawing surprising and innovative conclusions for ourselves. As a positive emotion, feeling curious expands our thinking.[19] And a bonus: activities that broaden attention also increase creative thinking.[20]

We need to make specific plans that lead to achieving our overarching eating and exercise goals. That's a given. But we also need to remember that, due to circumstances we could not have envisioned when we made the plan, we may not be able to stick to that *exact* plan. Keeping the door open to other possibilities at choice points can reduce stress and cultivate success.[21] But, just like I tell my clients, every once in a while we bump up against a choice point on a day where no perfect *imperfect* options or workable alternatives exist. In those instances, intentionally choosing to forgo your plan in its entirety might be the *right* choice *at that moment*, even if it's not a Joy Choice. Keep in mind that *you're* the only one who knows what you need, and remember to always be self-compassionate at those times too.

We always need to keep in mind that the true value of *any* choice is always determined by the context of other options and needs.[22] This chapter, we focused on the importance of context, opening your options, and playing with the possibilities through flexible thinking, fun, and curiosity—all within the specific circumstances of that moment and day. The next chapter explores the science and methods behind increasing the value of your healthy eating and exercise decisions in fundamental ways, helping you tilt the odds in favor of picking your Joy Choice.

Remember: The key to success is accepting that although our underlying goal remains steady, our plans will inevitably be challenged. And knowing that when we come to choice points, we are well prepared and actually eager to play with the possibilities that take us to our Joy Choice.

eleven

CHOOSE JOY: SUPPORTING INHIBITION

YOU MUST BE KIDDING!" SAID MARK. "I CAN HONESTLY SAY I WILL *NEVER* stop trying to lose weight." Mark's challenge came immediately after I suggested that he stop focusing on weight loss in order to develop a new, positive relationship with eating and exercise that would make self-control less effortful and meals more enjoyable.

"Mark," I explained, "I'm not proposing that you stop wanting to lose weight. What I *am* suggesting is that to develop the new positive associations with eating and exercise that are needed to support lasting changes, you'll need to press pause on primarily focusing on weight loss. Just for now."

This notion always seems to take people by surprise—not only clients, but professionals such as personal trainers whose job description includes helping people "get fit" and lose weight. I hear the same concern *100 percent of the time*, and it goes something like this: "But my clients are coming to me to lose weight. How can I tell them that we are not going to do that?" Mind you, their concern is valid, as are the concerns of their clients and my clients. But I assure you there is a logic to this seeming madness. It begins with the persuasive power of how we think about and frame our intended eating and exercise choices, the resulting experiences and memories they create, and ultimately whether we are able to achieve our overarching, long-term goal. So, just for now, as you read this chapter, I'm going to ask you, too, to press pause and imagine a mindset not in service of "losing weight" or "getting in shape" but in service of creating and living in a whole new world in which you actually enjoy eating in better ways and desire to exercise and be more active.

BEFORE YOU ENTER

Another client, Erin, reacting from a lifetime of emotionally painful experiences with sports and exercise—on the playground, in school, in the gym—literally snorted with derision when I suggested the possibility that being physically active could actually *feel good*. Except for the snort, I wasn't surprised by her reaction because I'd heard variations of it for decades. I told Erin what I will tell you: a growing body of research indicates that despite a rocky personal history, we *can* develop the new positive relationships with exercise and healthy eating that are a key part of achieving lasting change.

When I present this idea to my clients and to the clinicians I train, a few are intrigued and want to learn more, but most of them waste no time in letting me know how they feel. Lifelong struggles with body issues intertwined with eating and exercise leave many people feeling not only demoralized but cynical about the prospect of actually feeling good when they make healthy choices, and doubtful that they could ever develop a truly positive relationship with food and physical activity. Snorting is just one way people express how suspect and frankly impossible the idea of *choosing joy* is when it applies to healthier eating and exercise.

They have good reasons for feeling this way, and you may too. Based on years of bad experiences with exercise and eating endeavors, it's no surprise that we'd be skeptical that we could actually *look forward* to exercise, or that eating in healthier ways has anything to do with joy. It's human nature to avoid those past negative experiences that are embedded in our long-term memories, and go in the exact opposite direction.

This makes the idea of shifting our exercise and eating patterns even more challenging to consider. Why go to the gym when you already know it will just make you feel self-conscious? Why force yourself to eat an arugula salad when you know how comforted mac and cheese will make you feel? It makes me feel good too. I get why the concept of *choosing joy* when it comes to leaving the coziness of the couch or avoiding the enveloping warmth of foods we love—and having that joy be about doing something like working out or eating greens—may seem incomprehensible and maybe even downright crazy.

But when we step outside of the typical behavior change story we see something surprising. This new frame shows us that healthy eating and exercise don't have to involve the teeth-gritting, brute-force type of control we've been trying to exert for so long.

RETHINKING "SELF-CONTROL"

I had an epiphany about "self-control" when our new insurance agent, Kris, emailed me at the end of the day to say that she needed my credit card number to initiate the policy. Motivated to finalize this laborious process, and even more to just get this task off my crowded to-do list, I immediately responded asking her to call me right now so I could read her my card number because I felt uncomfortable emailing it. Instead of calling, however, she emailed right back with a request: "Good idea! Can I ring you tomorrow? I'm just about to leave for an exercise class."

Oh, the irony. I had wanted to check that call off *my* list. Yet I had to admit to myself that I coach individuals every day to protect their priorities—to do the very thing Kris had done! I couldn't help but be impressed and pleased by her quick response and purposeful ease. Rather than fall into the trap of accommodating my needs, she politely but firmly protected her planned class from being potentially derailed by what in my mind would take less than sixty seconds, but which in reality could have prevented her from leaving the office in time.

Did Kris just have great self-control? Maybe, but let's go a little deeper.

When we spoke later, I asked Kris why she had been so motivated to get to the gym. Her response says it all: "I just don't feel as good when I don't exercise and that negatively influences everything else that I do. So, for me, getting to the gym is essential." Kris's choice shows how effortless our exercise and eating choices can be when they are in service of something that is deeply compelling to us. In popular culture we tend to think of choices that keep us sticking to our eating and exercise plans as pure and simple "self-control." But this lauded ability also overlaps with the executive function formally called *inhibition* or *inhibitory control*. Inhibition helps us control our attention, choices, thoughts, and emotions to override a strong internal impulse or external lure so as to protect a goal we value and are striving to achieve.[1] But when it comes to eating and exercise, we don't say, "I really need to inhibit better." We say, "I need more self-control" or "If only I had more willpower." And the internal voice that says this generally sounds beaten down rather than energized.

The ability to control and inhibit ourselves has received way more attention—in this book, and in life—than the other two primary executive functions we are focusing on, working memory and flexible thinking. That's not because it *is* more important, but because self-control has basically been overinflated and billed as the hero of the behavior change story—the strict enforcer we need to restrict our impulses and keep us from our temptations. Yet by now, we've seen that self-control on its own can be overrated, and that even *wanting* more self-control can do more harm than good.[2]

When we overvalue our ability to inhibit our impulses, we put too much of our focus on a singularly controlling need. This can not only thwart our autonomy, it takes us in exactly the *wrong* direction. We get entrenched: The more we try to *force* ourselves to make a choice, the further down the rebellious mindset and self-sabotage rabbit hole we go, reinforcing our feeling that we just don't have enough "self-control" and undermining our ability to resist then and in the future. This diverts our attention from what *could have been helpful* and sets us up for failure. Worse, it's *exhausting*, depleting the very energy that could have helped our executive functions to actually function.

So, Kris got it right. She didn't need to *control* herself or *force* anything because she had a vision that she valued for her well-being and greater life context, and she gracefully, politely, and firmly protected it from harm. Kris did this by deploying an established strategy called *goal shielding*.[3]

GOAL SHIELDING: THE WONDER WOMAN EFFECT

I like the term goal shielding for a couple of reasons. Shielding, like inhibition, isn't weighted down by the psychic baggage of trying to *control* ourselves. It is also self-explanatory: we shield—or protect—our plans from that which could derail them. What an empowering concept! And a fine example of reframing.

When I think about goal shielding, an image of Wonder Woman crossing her arms over her chest and using her awesome bracelets to protect herself always pops into my mind. Notice she's not trying to *control* herself; she's using her abilities to *protect* herself and the things she most values. Things that she *wants to* protect. The effect is powerful, yet effortless, which puts Wonder Woman on the cutting edge of science.

When clients and professionals learn about this more empowering vision for protecting their goals, they always ask me whether there are any apps or programs that can help boost *their* inhibition. The answer is yes *and* no.

DOES INHIBITION TRAINING WORK?

The general logic behind inhibition training is that people can be trained to override and inhibit their impulses, preventing them from succumbing to tempting foods after these trainings. That sounds like a noble idea, but there's more to this story.

A common method of computer-based inhibition training is called *go/no-go*.[4] This type of training is based on the logic that you can learn to inhibit yourself by repeatedly practicing inhibiting. The trainings work like this: You receive prompts that you try to respond to as quickly as you can (often by tapping a computer) when you see a *go* stimulus (e.g., apple, broccoli), and *not responding* (by not tapping the key) when you see a *no-go* stimulus (e.g., French fries, cheesecake). The idea is that, with enough practice, your inhibitory response will become automatic, or "second nature."

Simple. But does it work? In the lab, sure.[5] But these improvements do not last once people leave the lab for the more complex world of real life. Confronted with the sight and scent of fresh, hot, crispy French fries, all that key-tapping success is no match for the mouth-watering memory you have of the last time you ate fries. To be fair, these types of trainings are still in their infancy.[6] But considering the true daily challenges and decision traps we face, these types of lab-based inhibition trainings might be "no-gos" for the many of us who are ready to take charge of our choices once and for all.

Rather than focusing on how to better inhibit or control ourselves, imagine what we could achieve if we turned this situation on its head. What if we turned our attention to what we *want* at our *deepest level*—beyond some number on the scale that we've been trying to achieve for years, beyond "getting fit," beyond a vague desire to "be healthier"—and go after *that?*

VALUE-BASED DECISION MAKING

You've already read about some of the findings from a focus group study of high-active versus low-active exercisers that I conducted with my coleaders, Drs. Heather Patrick and April Oh, and other esteemed colleagues, funded by the National Cancer Institute.[7] But our study was actually about something much bigger.

Our primary research question related to how people's greater life values and daily priorities influence their physical activity participation. What we found went straight to the heart, showing that the participants who were regularly active discussed physical activity as being congruent with their core identity and life goals. Being physically active supported their sense of autonomy, competence, and connection with others. It appeared to connect to who they were (and valued being) at the deepest level.

In contrast, low-active participants' comments did not suggest that they viewed physical activity as a way to support their greater values or daily priorities. On the contrary, they discussed physical activity in ways that suggested resentment and dread. They had unrealistic expectations about how exercise could reshape their bodies and perfectionistic beliefs about how much exercise they *should be* doing. Not surprisingly, many framed physical activity as a way to lose weight, felt an aversion to doing it, and judged themselves negatively for their lack of success.

These findings align with the experiences I've had with my coaching clients and a lot of research: A focus on weight loss when making changes in eating and exercise gets them all tangled up with complicated, negative experiences, which in turn motivates us to either *avoid* or *rebel* against them. In stark contrast to that self-rejecting roller coaster, when we learn to affirm our sense of self and what we most value *through* our exercise and eating choices, it doesn't just drive consistent decisions but also creates an actual *desire* for making them.[8] That is, *we want to stay consistent and we do.*

I don't know if this idea is familiar or surprising to you, or whether you feel skeptical that this is even possible. But to really understand the power of explicitly seeing healthy eating and exercise in service of our identity *and* the important people and projects in our lives, we need to step back and talk about what science shows *most drives* us as human beings; what makes us feel happy and successful and what brings true meaning and purpose to our lives.

Referred to by some as "value-based choice,"[9] the latest neuroscience helps explain the underlying mechanism for how our values and sense of identity motivate ongoing decision making that favors healthier eating and consistent physical activity. Our brain-based reward system is set up to generally desire things we like and find meaningful. In general, we choose things based on what we *anticipate* will be rewarding and valuable to us. So, when our choices bring us closer to who we want to be (in other words, are congruent with our identity, and what we value), this makes these choices inherently and deeply rewarding—not just in a heartfelt way, but by actually increasing activation deep within the brain regions that track the value we give things.[10]

Emily Falk, PhD, director of the University of Pennsylvania's Communication Neuroscience Lab, conducts research on this topic. Her work suggests that helping people see health-related communications as self-relevant and valuable—what is called self-affirming—is associated with greater activity in brain-based reward networks and also participation in healthy behavior.[11]

She used her own life as an example.[12] "I run to de-stress," she said. "I've never really thought of myself as a fast runner or even wanted to be a fast runner. But when my siblings encouraged me to get faster so I could keep up with them, it shifted my value calculation for running faster—going from something that seemed painful and pointless to something that had social value (being able to spend more time with them). My brother also suggested that because I was an academic, I already had the mental skills to train—a key part of research is doing the work now to achieve a later goal. He helped me view running faster as something that *is* congruent with my identity. In the brain, self-relevance and social relevance are two key inputs into our calculation of how valuable any given choice is to us. Finding those bridges between self-relevance, social relevance, and value for any small choice in the moment makes it possible to achieve our bigger goals in the future."

Just as Falk personally discovered with her own running, and I've seen time and again with my clients, a recently published study suggests that people *can be taught* to consider their healthy eating goals as part of their identity, and when they do, they make healthier eating choices and even perceive their eating goals as easier to pursue.[13]

Here's the exciting takeaway from this latest science: When the exercise and eating goals *we* have selected (as opposed to those that have been imposed on us by society or others) align with our core values, needs, and priorities, they become integrated into and a natural affirming part of who we are. This in turn increases the value proposition for making choices that favor healthy eating and regular exercise. Because we no longer feel that we *should* make these choices, our internal conflicts with them are gone or greatly reduced, and so now we *want* to make them and make them more effortlessly.[14]

But this raises an important question that I am often asked: Can we still drive our healthy eating and exercise choices if we do want to lose weight?

WEIGHT LOSS: IT'S COMPLICATED

As we've discussed throughout the book, weight loss as the primary reason for a behavior change is a complex, troubling, and painful issue for many. Tangled inextricably with healthy eating and exercise, it is a tender issue to address and a real conundrum.

On the one hand, we do want to eat better and be more active, and we believe that many things in our lives would be better if we lost weight. On the other hand, research suggests that *shoulds*, shame, self-deprecation, antipathy, Rebellion, and Perfection are born from coupling our lifestyle changes with striving to lose weight. *These negative forces are fierce opponents to lasting change.* And here's where the rubber meets the road: If we can't achieve lasting change, we *also* can't achieve any sustainable outcome, regardless of the goal.

I was talking about this issue the other day with my old friend Evan from graduate school. He had become a clinical psychologist whose practice emphasized health coaching and lifestyle change. He told me about a recent lecture he'd attended on weight stigma and bias where the speaker had discussed how emotionally damaging and harmful they are for mental health. The speaker also noted that when people try to change their health behaviors *in order to lose weight*, exercising and healthy eating get twisted up with this greater stigma, easily converting eating and exercise into *self*-stigmatizing behaviors that can cause inner conflicts and demotivation; the very things that derail our intended decisions.

Evan asked me how he could work with his patients to help unravel lifestyle behaviors from these decision-disrupting forces. "Think about it this way," I said, "there are no absolutes. But the reality is that there's generally been only *one* behavior change story and it's socialized our society to have the same beliefs and associations with trying to eat better and exercise more. And they are centrally focused on losing weight."

I explained that not everyone is plagued by these complexities and conflicts associated with losing weight. But *when they are explicitly in service of losing weight*, it's all too easy for healthy eating and exercise to convert from what should just be life-enhancing into behaviors that evoke or exacerbate shame, self-loathing, and similar negative emotions that may have been carried around for years.

"Look," I continued, "even if we want to lose weight for medically important or other compelling reasons, this weight loss *goal* can still be wrapped up with these demotivating and self-rejecting forces, getting all tangled up with healthy eating and physical activity. In this scenario, there's zero degrees of separation between those entrenched negative experiences and healthy eating and exercise."

Evan was shaking his head. "Yeah," I agreed. "It's really complicated."

The value of any choice we make is always determined by the context of other options but also *by the costs* that come from making that choice.[15] Better eating and exercise that are twisted up with *shoulds* or self-rejection reflect psychological costs that would, in turn, devalue these behaviors (unconsciously and consciously),[16] likely motivating us to *not* choose them at choice points.

I told Evan, "The bottom line is, it's hard to make sustainable changes in healthy eating and exercise if we are striving to lose weight with these associations—there's virtually nothing sustaining about negativity, resentment, and shame." The irony is undeniable.

I suggested to Evan that he might talk with his patients about all of these issues, with the ultimate goal of self-reflection; helping them explore their past traps but also cultivating curiosity about the ways in which they could create a new behavior change story and finally learn how to achieve the lasting change they've been after.

The Joy Choice aims to help resolve this knotty problem by helping you better understand the research behind this challenging issue but also the compelling science pointing to the solution. It's not weight loss per se that's the problem, it's the complexities that are often lurking underneath. Sometimes, to liberate exercise and better eating from these harmful meanings, some clients find it helpful to ask themselves what their *underlying* motivation is for losing weight and why they care about *that*. This line of questioning can help identify the *often concealed* real value of losing weight (such as having more energy, staying healthy to care for others, feeling better more generally). This, in turn, lets them reframe their thinking and put their lifestyle behaviors in service of that deeper reason. But other clients decide to make a clean break and ditch their weight-loss goal, freeing them up to discover another goal that more deeply resonates in self-supporting, positive ways.

RECLAIMING WHAT'S YOURS: YOUR EXPERIENCES

Can exercise and healthy eating really feel good on a sustainable basis? Yes, they can. But we have to get there first. Here's how it worked with my client Ben.

"Okay, Ben," I said. "Let's try an experiment with eating this week. How about we toss out all of the 'rules' you told me you've learned to follow and let yourself eat whatever you want this week. But there's one catch: you only eat something *after* you tune into your body and notice what it's feeling, what your body seems to want. Then, try to stay mindful of your experiences *while* you eat and afterward. Does that seem doable?"

Ben was initially quite doubtful. Like so many logically fear, he was also very worried that he'd go overboard with eating and not be able to stop. I suggested that even if that worst-case scenario occurred, it would only be for a week. After considering this, and realizing he'd never tried this strategy before, his curiosity overcame some of his worry, and he agreed to try it until our next session, one week later.

"So, how did your experiment go?" I asked the following week.

"Michelle, it was so weird to do this. The first day, I just had to keep remembering to pay attention to what I was doing. I'm not used to checking in with my body at all, so I was like, 'Are you hungry?' 'Are you full yet?' To be honest, at first it felt kind of embarrassing— partly by having to ask the questions, but also because I didn't feel anything. But after the first few days, I started to notice things were shifting a little. By midweek, I did start to feel new experiences with eating. I actually started to taste the food I ate, that was new!

"At lunch, I noticed that I definitely wanted a pizza," he continued, "but when I checked in with myself, I was surprised to learn that I only wanted two slices. Then, yesterday, something really crazy happened. My colleague at work was passing around a box of chocolate truffles. I started to reach for one automatically, because that's my weak spot, but then I remembered our deal. I stopped myself and paused to check in with myself. I couldn't believe what I noticed! I didn't actually *feel like* eating chocolate! Never in my life have I ever experienced anything like this, and I would have bet a lot of money against you if you'd suggested I would."

Ben credits his "ah-ha" moment with the chocolate truffles for transforming his relationship with food. He continued the experiment for the rest of the week and beyond, continuing to *learn more about what foods actually felt like*—while he was eating, afterward, and even the next day.

This huge shift is pretty wild when you think about it: When we give ourselves permission to drop the rules and toss out the *shoulds*, it quiets the negative noise, clears out the distraction, and creates the space to really notice how we *feel* with and from our food choices. We start to actually taste the food, and sometimes discover that it doesn't taste as good as we had previously thought before eating in this more mindful way. Liberated from following rules that he only wanted to rebel against, Ben was free to start using his own body as the sensor it always had the potential to be. Like other clients, he started to feel a greater sense of agency over his eating choices, and made intentional choices rather than rebellious ones. He also stopped thinking about food all of the time like he used to.

Becoming *aware* of our own personal traps and replacing restrictive rules with a more intuitive approach to eating has the potential to make inner struggle less relevant because the struggle has been *replaced* by curiosity and appreciation. And this shift can liberate us beyond the menu. It also engenders a deeper sense of trust about our greater wisdom and decision making ability.

This might sound overly simplistic or unbelievable, but I assure you it is neither. This transformative shift in thinking and decision making reflects the cutting-edge science about the mechanisms deep in our bodies and minds that help us *learn* how to reduce craving-related eating and learn to enjoy healthier foods. Judson Brewer, MD, PhD, director of Research and Innovation at Brown University's Mindfulness Center, leads a program of research that addresses this very issue.[17] His and other mindfulness-based research suggests that when we notice how we feel in the moment of eating, we are better able to understand the *full set* of experiences that accompany eating something delicious, including potentially negative ones too.

Here's how it works: When we have a *heightened awareness* of the experiences we feel in our bodies, it helps us *learn* the true value from our eating choices, not just how it tastes going down. For example, if we eat too much pizza, it will likely also come with costs in the moment or afterward, including feeling overfull, maybe guilt, regret, or more.[18] This process helps us learn the *real* value that comes from eating too much pizza (hint: It's decreased!). This updated valuation gets logged into our memories so the next time we choose how much to eat, this experience becomes a future reference and influence. But this learning process isn't just for food—it also applies to physical activity.[19]

My client Trisha is a great example of this. When we started our work, she'd told me that for years, she'd started running with her standard New Year's resolution to take off the baby weight she'd put on with her two children. But as she told me more than once, "I hate running. I keep trying because I think that's the quickest way for me to lose weight. But it leaves me so tired and resentful, I usually quit after just a few weeks." In our work together, running was off the table because the way we learn lasting change in this new system necessitates that the physical activities we participate in feel positive in some way, or at the very least, not punishing. In fact, the research on this is quite clear. How we feel *during* exercise, not afterward, is what predicts whether we stay the course.[20]

She got another job, and life got hectic, and our work stopped. But a few years later, she emailed me to catch up and that's when I received a surprise! "Michelle, you are never going to believe this, but now I love running and do it every day. It makes me feel so happy." When I asked what changed, she said, "Well, things at my job got really stressful and one day the stress was so high that I was about to combust. For some reason, I decided to go running. That run felt completely different than any run before. It helped release that stress, and I felt more grounded afterward, like I could handle the work situation better. Ever since, my running experiences have been so positive. I've found it easy to develop new friendships with other women who like to run, and it's become a very important part of my life."

As Trisha's story shows, the experience doing the same activity (in her case, running) transformed, from a strong negative to a strong positive, once she changed her primary reason for running from losing weight to relieving stress. Aligning with the science, her new positive experiences (stress release, feeling grounded) and meanings (friendship, community) instilled new memories; she *learned* to like and want these experiences, and she is still going (running) strong.

Positive experiences are important in driving the healthy eating and exercise decisions that change our behavior.[21] We can cultivate them on our own or get assistance doing it. (I designed a clinician tool specifically for them to guide patients in this process, and you can find it in Appendix B.)

The transformations experienced by Trish and Ben reflect the learning process that happens when we increase the value of our lifestyle choices by redesigning them to deliver more positive experiences and a heighted awareness of them. This learning process can occur in many different ways. But I've found it more easily happens within the context of a *new* purpose and meaning for healthy eating and exercise, one that affirms instead of rejects who we are, and that asks us to care about our preferences and how our bodies feel.

Here's a thought experiment that might take you right into the heart of the issue:

Take a moment to think about working out or following an eating plan that you started in order to lose weight or that your doctor strongly recommended for losing weight. Don't dwell on it; just close your eyes and quickly call up your past experiences, feelings, struggles, and memories. Then, check in with yourself: How does the idea about exercising feel right now? How desirable is that planned meal?

Now, let's take it in a different direction: Forget about losing weight, looking "better," or following doctor's orders. Instead, imagine that you are changing your eating or exercising *explicitly* in service of feeling better, of taking better *care of yourself*, and of being fully present and energized in service of your family, friends, professional goals, and community. Pause here for a moment to imagine what *that* feels like. Check in with yourself: Did that vision of eating better or exercising feel at all different than the first one? Most people say they *do* feel differently, at least somewhat more positive, grounded, or enlivened.

YOUR GREATER GOAL INFLUENCES YOUR EXECUTIVE FUNCTIONING

That was not just an exercise in "visioning." As you've learned, it reflects what emerging science suggests will help you better achieve lasting changes in eating and exercise. **We're talking about the same behaviors, transformed by putting them in service of a different goal.** This new framing also supports our executive functioning.

The new thinking about executive functions views them as a team that works *in service* of a specific goal, and of the beliefs, knowledge, norms, pressures, interests, and preferences related to that goal, rather than as stand-alone abilities that could be boosted in isolation from one another, through lab-based computer tasks or games.[22] And how could they not? Our motivation to protect our plan from a conflict through inhibiting it, as Kris did with my request for a call, or being motivated to play with the possibilities at a choice point is inextricably connected to our beliefs, knowledge, desires, and the pressures we experience in relation to exercising and healthy eating.

The good news is that when we use healthy eating and physical activity to *affirm* our identity and support our values and daily priorities, we solve problems better, even when we are stressed.[23] Having a deeply compelling goal we want to protect at a choice point helps mobilize our executive functions. It reducees the noise and inner conflicts that can tax our working memory, increasing its capacity and our ability to focus. And, with our meaningful aspiration in the forefront of our mind, we can more easily inhibit distractions and keep them at bay. In addition, we are more motivated to use flexible thinking: Do we inhibit and completely skip out on any of the treats, or are there other possibilities we could play with at this choice point that would better meet our full set of needs? Our executive functions better rally when they are explicitly in service of a goal that aligns with our identity and daily priorities versus one that we're motivated to rebel against.

At the beginning of the chapter, I asked you to experiment with pressing pause on any weight-loss goal you might have, to give you an opportunity to visit this new desirable world I'm suggesting exists for healthy eating and exercise. I don't know where you've landed or if you've already un-paused. Regardless of your choice, I'm not suggesting that you ever stop striving to eat in healthier ways or become more active. Rather, based on past experience, common sense, and a lot of science, I do contend that you will become more successful making the consistent decisions that underlie lasting change *if you can put them in service of achieving a goal that explicitly asserts your worth, helps you feel your best, and serves your deepest values.*

When our eating and exercise choices affirm our sense of self, and our needs, priorities, and preferences, we no longer need to *control* ourselves because now we *want to* protect them. But this new behavior change story doesn't just support inhibition, it creates the stable and energizing driver of our full executive functioning team, making our choices more effortless. And that's what I call choosing joy.

THE JOY OF CHOOSING JOY

Joy means different things to different people, but I'd like to tell you what it means in the Joy Choice solution. Here, the ultimate purpose of choosing joy is to learn how to sustain ourselves through regular physical activity and better eating, and in so doing, to sustain our greater life values and daily priorities.

MY LIFE

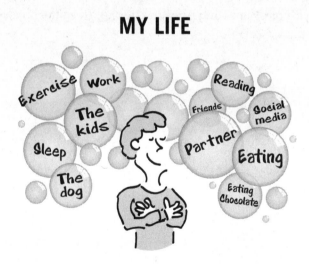

When we reframe physical activity and more thoughtful eating choices in this way, after a short while we begin to notice new rewards: we feel more positive and have more energy, and that helps us perform better as parents, partners, and professionals. We learn that our eating and exercise choices not only help us sustain ourselves, they sustain the other people and projects we care most about too.[24] When we learn to think in this integrative way, it helps increase the value of healthier eating and physical activity within our brain and within our day.[25] The more we engender and enjoy these positive rewards, the more motivated we are to keep striving to have them. This cycle results from the positive feedback loop of making healthy choices that we learn helps us feel more positive, giving us more energy and enthusiasm to tend to our most meaningful life areas. A self-sustaining cycle indeed!

Choosing joy doesn't mean that our eating and exercise plans won't face conflicts—in fact, they always will. So, in the next chapter, we turn our attention to the Joy Choice decision tool, POP!, to learn the how-tos of picking the perfect *imperfect* options that keep us consistent with our values and priorities, within this life-enhancing and self-sustaining cycle.

twelve

= POP! =

THE JOY CHOICE DECISION TOOL AND HOW TO USE IT

N ONE OF US HAS A CRYSTAL BALL. WE CAN'T KNOW WHAT'S COMING OUR way, but we do know that, like it or not, something will happen—occasionally, or predictably often—to disrupt our plans. The amount of unexpected things we encounter is directly proportional to the number of roles we inhabit in our daily lives. No wonder it's so hard for eating and exercise plans to survive.

To make it even more difficult, each of our life areas comes equipped not only with obligations (like picking the kids up from school, going to work in the morning, getting homework in on time), but with *should* expectations that complicate our plans on an emotional level:

Can I just forget about the gym and chill for a while?

Am I allowed to delegate cooking a meal to my partner when I'm trying to fit in a missed workout?

Will I look selfish if I skip the meeting for a walk?

Can I eat differently than my family?

Am I going to seem rude to my coworkers if I don't eat the treats they bring to work?

But consider that when it comes to the nonexercise and noneating parts of our lives, we generally *do* know how to find fifteen minutes to play catch with our kids before dinner, or take Mom to the doctor, or catch up on work for half an hour before bedtime, or fit in several two-minute quality partner check-ins throughout an otherwise busy day. We are grown-up children, moms and dads, siblings and friends, employees, professionals, and entrepreneurs. We know how to slice and dice our time and planning so we can juggle the meaningful bits and pieces of our lives and keep going.

We've already learned to do this because, well, it's necessary. We accept that these important life responsibilities are priorities that need to be sliced and diced to make them work. It's intuitive. Yet— and this is important—because of the old behavior change story, we didn't learn to think in this more fluid way about our lifestyle behaviors—even though they *also* have to survive in the same hubbub and complexity of our daily lives.

But we can learn to do the same thing with exercise and healthy eating that we do with our other life bits. The first trick is deciding that they are *equally worthy* of slicing and dicing as our other import-ant life areas. Then, we need to be able to give ourselves *permission* to slice and dice them in the same way.

No longer letting life burst our bubble, we learn to POP! our plan into usable parts through using the Joy Choice decision tool. By definition, the Joy Choice is the perfect *imperfect* option at a choice point that lets us slice and dice, doing something instead of nothing (regarding our eating and exercise plans). And at choice points that's really all we're after.

We've talked about the Joy Choice solution, and the sci-ence behind how its three strategies, Simplify, Play, and Choose

Joy, support our three primary executive functions at our choice points. And we've seen some examples of how the POP! decision tool works in clients' lives. Now, I'd like to formally introduce you to POP!; explain how it *embodies* Simplify, Play, and Choose Joy; and teach you how to use it when you come to choice points in your own life.

WHY WE POP!

There are a bunch of cool science-based reasons that POP! can help support our in-the-moment decision making.

POP! supports working memory: POP! is simple and easy to recall. As we discussed in the Simplify chapter, our working memory capacity is limited. We need to protect its precious space, keeping it free of distractions and TRAPs. We can support it through simple and engaging concepts like POP! that we can bring to mind at choice points, focusing our attention on the simple sequence of steps. In addition, the accompanying graphics help us visualize and encode the POP! steps,[1] making it easier to remember when we are thinking on our feet.

POP! supports flexible thinking: POP! embodies Play. It's *all about playfully* exploring options and possibilities, implicitly and explicitly supporting the cognitive flexibility that is fundamental to effective problem solving.

POP! supports inhibition: POP! helps us flip this tired conversation away from singularly needing to inhibit our impulses or *control* ourselves to a wider strategy that can help us achieve what we deeply *want* for ourselves, others, and the projects we care most about.

POP! lets us pick the perfect *imperfect* option: POP!'s ultimate objective is guiding us away from the dead end of either-or thinking and toward the Joy Choice, the perfect *imperfect* option that allows us to tend to our own self-care needs *and* meet the unanticipated needs of our day. In this way, we make the choices that keep us consistent, our golden ticket on the journey of lasting change.

Now, let's move on to how you can use POP! when you come up against challenges to your eating and exercise plans in your own life.

⇒POP!⇐

PAT'S STORY: A GUIDE TO POP!

Use Pat and Pat's exercise plan to guide yourself through the first two phases: Pre-POP! (your plan and your choice point) and POP! (the fun part!).

PRE-POP!

Generally, when we create plans for anything, including healthy eating and exercise, we make them with an assumption that they're good plans that will work. Otherwise, why bother? So this pre-POP! phase starts with the premise that you've got some kind of plan in place, whether you made it an hour, a few hours, days, or weeks in advance. Here's how it goes for Pat, who has used the POP! tool for a while now:

The Plan. *This is Pat's awesome exercise PLAN. It's perfect, and it seems easy to achieve: a thirty-minute workout at the gym after work. What could go wrong?*

Pat assumes that all of the other important parts of life that day—helping with the kids' homework, buying groceries, walking the dog, answering

MY EXERCISE PLAN

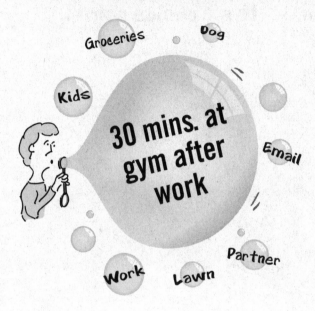

email, *finishing work—will easily find their place before and after that workout. But then the boss walks into Pat's office.*

The Unexpected Conflict = Choice Point! *Pat's boss announces that the timing of the big report, which had been due in two days, has been moved up. It is now due in one hour—end of day today. Ack! The work crisis looms, the gym plan looks doomed, and Pat automatically starts to head down Either-Or Road. But almost immediately, Pat's has a realization. "This isn't a conflict, I'm at a* **CHOICE POINT.**"

When we recognize we are facing a conflict, we learn to automatically cue up "choice point" in our minds, creating an automatic association that subsequently kicks our conscious thinking into gear. In contrast to conflicts disrupting the habit loop, **in the Joy Choice**

LIFE IS HAPPENING, CONFLICTS ARISE...
It's a choice point!

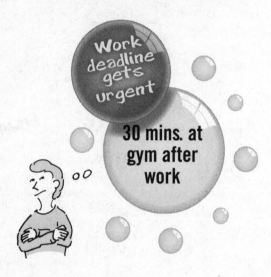

solution, conflict—*which is inevitable and unavoidable in life*—is what *engages* our executive functions, the mental prowess we need to successfully resolve this conflict. We can't stop having unexpected conflicts between life and our eating and exercise plans, *but we can change how we think and what we do at our choice points.*

Regardless of what the conflict is, what matters is that you recognize it as *your choice point*, creating your opportunity to choose.

POP! 1-2-3

POP! is a simple decision tool you can use to quickly sort through your options after challenges to your plan bring you face-to-face with a choice point. POP! snaps you out of your old automatic and unhelpful reactions and TRAPs, bringing your focus back to *this* moment so you can reclaim your freedom to choose what works best for your beautiful, complicated life and the people and things that live in it with you. The first thing to do is to recognize that while your original plan may be unworkable, all is not lost. It's time to POP! your plan.

*Pat, who has encountered choice points many times before, thinks, "This is an opportunity to pick the Joy Choice! Time to **POP!** my plan and see what I can come up with." And that's just what Pat does.*

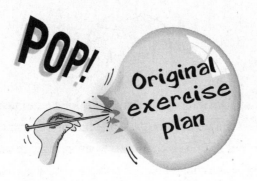

Pause
Open up your options and play
Pick the Joy Choice

POP! has three steps that are easy to recall in the moment you need them because they create the acronym you'll learn to remember, POP:

1. **P**ause
2. **O**pen up your options and play
3. **P**ick the Joy Choice

With the old plan gone, Pat runs through the three-step POP! process.

Step 1. Pause

<u>P</u>AUSE

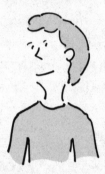

Ahh, the Pause. Quieting our breath and taking a moment to regroup is nothing new; the wisdom of *the pause* has been practiced for thousands of years. But its value is enormous when it comes to supporting our working memory at a choice point. Pausing and taking a few slow, calming breaths is a science-based winning strategy for our working memory.

- Slow breathing can *immediately* improve executive functioning performance.[2]
- Pausing to take a breath interrupts automatic thinking so we can name and release our TRAPs before they have the chance to pull us under.[3]
- Pausing establishes mindful awareness, so we can make intentional choices that best serve us and our lives.[4]
- Pausing lets us shift gears, refocus, and engage our executive functions.[5]

In the Joy Choice, one benefit of the Pause is to give ourselves the opportunity to identify any TRAPs that are close by.

Pat's typical TRAP is Accommodation, especially when it comes to prioritizing work over other needs. Pat might have completely tossed out the exercise plan, lost in thought about this new urgent timing need. But not this time! Pat said, "Pat, you can do this. You can figure this out."

When we call ourselves by name, we engage what's called "distanced self-talk." This seemingly simple tactic immediately puts us into the observer role, creating the strategic distance that helps us get perspective. Research by University of Michigan psychologist Ethan Kross suggests this strategy is helpful for kids and adults, and is also associated with making healthier choices.[6] Getting some distance helps us understand that while we *have* these feelings, thoughts, and experiences, we *are not* our feelings or our experiences. We can then step back, observe, and choose with awareness and intention.

Step 2. Open up your options and play

Some of my clients are excited by the idea of playing with the possibilities, while others express concern about their ability to "open up and play." To them it sounds vague and limitless, and intimidating to even think about. If this similarly feels overwhelming to you, I've got some tips to get you through.

Choice points are all about logistics, managing plans and resources—in this case, time, activities, place, food choices. When you POP! your plan, you are opening up your logistical alternatives.

It's easier to find something when we need it if we organize it in a specific place. You can think of POP! as an "organizer" for storing, accessing, and considering other options and possibilities. POP! is also a decision system that makes your choice point more manageable through easy questions you can ask yourself. For example, "What else can I do or eat instead? How much time do I actually have? When else today might I be able to make work?" There's no need to stress with this task because the goal is just to generate ideas and options, suspending any judgment about their value. The key word here is *generate*, not evaluate.

Pat's been through this before, so it doesn't take long to play with the possibilities at hand. Go to the gym for a shorter time—maybe fifteen minutes, given the time it takes to get there and change clothes? Walk with the family after dinner for thirty minutes? Pat could already hear the kids grumbling about that one. Dance to some energizing music? Oh, where did that idea come from?!

OPEN UP YOUR OPTIONS
AND PLAY

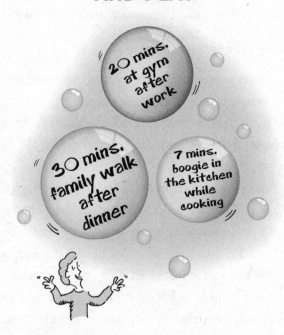

Look at your options. Which ones work best with your real life today? Which ones make you grit your teeth just to think about?

Which ones make you breathe a little easier just thinking about? Now throw out any remaining *shoulds* and get genuinely curious about how the different possibilities might work. Be open to considering something you've never tried before, which is what Pat just did.

Feeling optimistic that some type of workout is still on the horizon, Pat is ready for Step 3.

Step 3. Pick the Joy Choice

Now you're ready to Pick the Joy Choice. Here's what Pat decided.

After playing with the possibilities and considering what would work best, Pat realized that dancing with headphones on was actually the easiest and most enjoyable option. And it could be combined with dinner prep, so no real extra time was needed. Waiting for water to boil would be much more fun if dancing were involved! And even just seven minutes of that activity would bring a welcome burst of happy energy after a hard day.

<u>P</u>ICK THE J<u>O</u>Y C<u>H</u>OICE

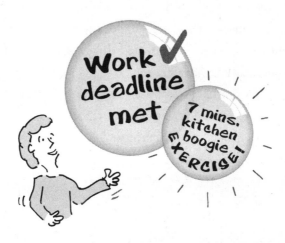

How do *you* feel about Pat's Joy Choice? I know that changing our thinking about this can be a tough nut to crack (because some of my clients have made this very clear!). Your first reaction might be to doubt the value of doing *any* physical activity for only seven minutes, or even outside of the gym, for that matter. Or if you're thinking about the Joy Choice in regard to healthy eating, you may initially think that it isn't worth considering alternative options at choice points if they don't explicitly line up with an ideal. But the research on the benefits of being flexible with eating and exercise plans strongly suggests otherwise, as does my real-world experience coaching people.

By using the POP! decision tool and picking the Joy Choice, we move beyond old, ineffective, and even self-sabotaging ways of approaching eating and exercise that have never gotten us where we actually want to go. We banish *shoulds* and put *ourselves* in charge, we continually reaffirm our own self-worth and align ourselves with our core values and daily priorities. And—bottom line for meeting our eating and exercise objectives—we ensure that we keep making the consistent, in-the-moment choices that keep us in sync with ourselves and the people and things we value most. Oh, and also? POP! isn't just helpful, it's fun too!

What happens after you've POP!ed? Now, you get to assess how things went. Afterward, Pat assessed this boogie-based Joy Choice, was quite pleased with how it turned out, and made a mental note to remember it for another choice point. But even if you are not totally pleased with your Joy Choice as Pat was, that's okay; *it's all experience we put toward learning lasting change*, which is where we're headed to right now in the last chapter.

thirteen

LEARNING LASTING CHANGE

LASTING CHANGE IS POWERED BY CONSISTENTLY MAKING THE IN-THE-moment choices that are aligned with our core self, help us feel our best, and fuel what matters most. But we don't actually *achieve* lasting change—we *learn* it.

We began this book talking about the pros and cons of *habit learning*: making our eating and exercise choices automatic, rote, and reflexive, with no need for thought. This type of learning works better for some people and for simple, routine actions like putting our keys in the same place after work or flossing our teeth before bedtime. But for many of us, despite planning and schedules, our days are usually far from simple or routine.

Automatic habits reflect inflexible and rigid strategies that are driven by past outcomes.[1] They *inhibit* the very psychological flexibility and creative problem solving we need when we bump up against novel challenges,[2] like choice points. If habit learning is not a good fit when we want to achieve lasting changes in eating and exercise, then what is? It's the very *opposite*.

In contrast to the stable contexts and cues habit learning needs to stick, learning lasting change within *The Joy Choice* assumes an ever-changing complex life that requires ongoing learning. And this calls for conscious and intentional strategizing—that is, thinking.

THINKING ABOUT YOUR THINKING

The Joy Choice invites you to *think about* how you think about your healthy eating and exercise projects, plans, and goals. No, I didn't accidentally write "think about" twice. Science has a word for this type of thinking: *metacognition*,[3] which simply (and, I think, delight-fully) means "thinking about your own thinking."[4]

Metacognition is when we use our conscious minds in the *most strategic ways*: to have a keen awareness of the challenges that tend to arise, and of how eating and exercise choices make us feel. Metacognition allows us to evaluate the results from our choice-point-related decision making by asking ourselves questions like: *Did it deliver the intended benefits to me and my day? Could I be more play-ful the next time I POP!?* We can't change our choice patterns and behaviors in lasting ways if we don't learn to think differently about them. And we can only learn to change our thinking about eating and exercise to be more adaptive if we begin to monitor how we think about it!

Metacognition is the conscious and tactical thinking that we need to learn lasting change. But if the idea of learning lasting change through metacognition seems daunting, consider that it just reflects the easy-to-use process that you've already been benefiting from throughout your lifetime. Simply, metacognition is becoming *an observer* of ourselves.

We do it naturally, for example, when we cook a new recipe we find online. We follow the steps, eat the meal, and then shift into the observer role to assess how it turned out. Does it taste the way we expected? The next time we try the recipe, we think about how it tasted and assess what specifically we didn't like (it had too much salt for our taste) and decide to tweak the recipe, reducing the amount of salt. After we eat, we assess our experience. Pretty good! Maybe, next time, we'll add some other ingredients and see what happens. We learned how to cook this new dish, not just by doing it, but by becoming an observer of our experience. This allowed us to reflect on it and identify what we liked, what worked or didn't, and what we might want to do differently next time.

We do this with *everything* we want to learn: becoming a better parent, playing an instrument, writing a book, nurturing friendships…Life is all about learning through metacognition! Learning how to stay the course in healthy eating and exercise involves using this same self-observing perspective, engaging our consciousness so we can monitor and course correct as needed.

Since you began reading *The Joy Choice*, in fact, you have been on a metacognitive journey of learning lasting change! You became this self-observer in Chapter 1, when you assessed whether you were more like a habiter or unhabiter. Then, as you read across the four TRAP chapters (Temptation, Rebellion, Accommodation, and Perfection), you were thinking about the relevance of each one in your own life. Metacognition is what has let you evaluate whether the beliefs, goals, and frames in the old behavior change story delivered as promised; and if not, it let you consider how you could apply these insights to create a new story that works better for you.

For example, it may be that when you first Pause at a choice point and consider your TRAPs, you become aware of a flood of negative thoughts: *This is ridiculous, I don't know how to do this, why would I expect things to turn out differently now,* and on and on. Metacognition lets you notice that thought, label it as unhelpful, let it go, and move on. Even if the negative thought derails your POP! process this time, *just bringing awareness to what took it down* helps you anticipate, get prepared, and strategize how to get past it at the next choice point. This is metacognition at work.

Beyond this tactical application, metacognition helps us learn the real rewards of picking the Joy Choice, feeling our best, and aligning our actions with our sense of self and values. Every time we pick the Joy Choice, we further integrate healthy eating and physical activity with who we are at our deepest level. This creates an ever-expanding positive feedback loop we can notice, name, and celebrate. And if no such loop exists, then we can use our metacognitive skills to figure out what's amiss and use those insights to course correct.

Metacognition is considered essential within the science of learning[5] because it is the process through which we *teach ourselves* what we need to know. It reflects a discovery process that helps us learn through doing and invites us to think *for* ourselves and *about* ourselves, as both thinker, learner, and change agent. And what could be better than that?

THE JOY CHOICE PATH: RETHINKING, REFRAMING, AND REIMAGINING

Throughout this book, you've been asked to rethink choice points, not as stressors or roadblocks but as opportunities to choose the perfect *imperfect* options that underlie lasting success. Then, you learned how our executive functions evolved to help us do things we've never done before. You were asked to consider how you could start using this new information to confront novel challenges, play with possibilities and options through the POP! decision tool, and ultimately Pick the Joy Choice—the in-the-moment choice that tends to your needs and lets you replenish your resources for what matters most that day.

We often need assistance starting a new change in behavior, and we look to books, health coaches, programs, or apps. But to *close the gap* between gaining momentum and maintaining change, what we want necessitates something larger and more personal. We need a new way of thinking that guides us to be open and curious about ourselves and our possibilities, and inspires us to keep learning how to make the consistent decisions that underlie lasting change. This is the Joy Choice in all its glory. This graphic shows us exactly how all of its bits, pieces, and parts fit together.

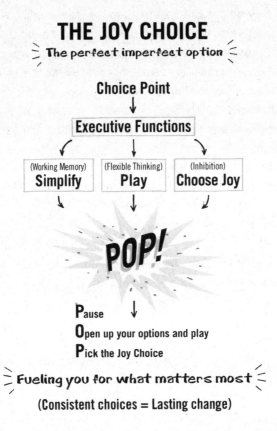

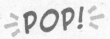

DAVID'S POP!
REALIZATION

Learning lasting change is the tactical thinking we use to successfully navigate from choice point to choice point. Let's look at how these ideas can play out through a new POP! story.

David and his partner, Leslie, decided to save some money by dropping their gym memberships. They already had some weights and a perfectly good exercise bike in their finished basement. They decided to add a rowing machine, which they had loved using at the gym.

Excited to begin, David set it up and the next morning before work he went into his basement to row for ten minutes while listening to his favorite podcast. He noticed he felt *okay* rowing, but something was missing and he was glad when it was over. He did this a few times that first week but started to notice a general feeling of "meh" (metacognition!) when he contemplated rowing. He wondered if the timing of his rowing was the problem, so he experimented with rowing after work for ten minutes the next time.

At the end of the week, on his way downstairs to row after work, he had a sudden, overwhelming realization: He did not want to be in the basement (metacognition!)! The rowing machine at the gym had been in a big room, near a sunny window. But his basement was completely different, small and a little dark. He thought he *should* be motivated—they had just bought that new machine! But he recognized this unproductive thought as he saw Perfection's shadow approaching, with Rebellion following right behind. Fortunately, David suddenly made the connection, naming the choice point he was at.

David knew what he had to do (metacognition!): POP! his plan.

LIFE IS HAPPENING, CONFLICTS ARISE...

It's a choice point!

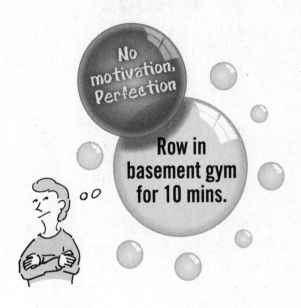

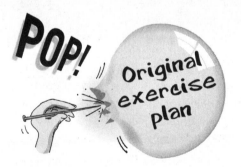

Pause
Open up your options and play
Pick the Joy Choice

1. Pause

PAUSE

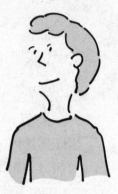

David took a breath. *I see you, Perfection and Rebellion!* He named those two TRAPs (metacognition!) before they could pull him under, and moved quickly to *Open up his options and play.*

2. **O**pen up your options and play

The first thing he did was quickly think through the What Else? When? And How Much? He knew he might have to slice and dice like he would other life areas to make it work.

He recognized that he had to stick with *now*, there was no other option today. When he considered *what else* he could do, riding the bike was even less appealing than rowing. But walking outside (sunshine! fresh air!) was calling his name, so much so that he decided to forgo his planned predinner email catch-up session to walk for forty-five minutes. This gave him plenty of time to enjoy the beautiful fall afternoon before it was time to make dinner with his family.

OPEN UP YOUR OPTIONS AND PLAY

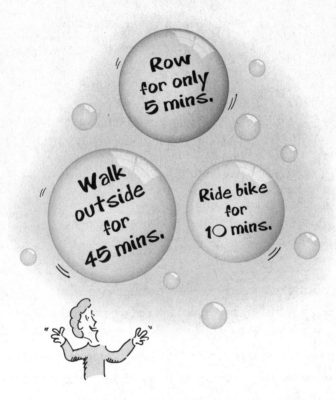

3. Pick the Joy Choice

He easily *Picked the Joy Choice*. Once he thought about how great it would feel to be outside, it was no contest. He realized that the forty-five-minute walk would lift his mood and start his night off great (metacognition!). David even invited one of his kids to come with him and ride her scooter. Much better than going it alone in the basement!

Pick the Joy Choice

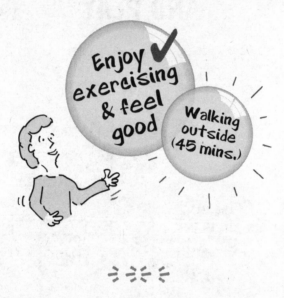

Not being motivated to follow through on a plan is among the most common challenges people face. *But it's actually just another type of choice point.* I help my clients learn that when they feel "unmotivated" it is a smokescreen for what's *really* going on: Typically, this is due to not actually wanting to do or liking the activity they had planned to do or the eating plan they had created. In David's case, it wasn't the actual physical activity that was unpleasant, it was the *context* of the exercise (his basement) that created it. Whatever the cause of "feeling unmotivated," this gut-level inclination or memory (remember the ART theory of physical inactivity and exercise in the Temptation chapter?) acts as an internal *stop sign* that is hard to ignore. But when we open ourselves to thinking about *how we are thinking about it* (metacognition!) we gain the insight we need to easily turn these situations around.

Through metacognition, David learned he wouldn't be active if he felt that he *should* work out in the basement, but he also learned that he would be active—and joyfully so—when his activity allowed him to be outside. He also realized that since Leslie enjoyed using the rowing machine, the expense was not a waste. Every so often, he asks himself whether he wants to row for only ten minutes instead of taking a much longer walk outside. But when David anticipates how these two different experiences will feel, despite the potential time savings, the walk winds up the winner.

Like David, when we gain awareness about our thinking and experiences, we are harnessing our consciousness and becoming our own best problem solvers. Humans learn best when we are actively engaged and exploring things that are personally meaningful to us and our lives.[6] The more you play with this process, the better you'll learn it. Please don't be daunted even if you think parts of it will be challenging! Like learning *anything in life*, it just takes time, practice, patience, and self-compassion. I encourage you to let go of expectations, let yourself enjoy and find meaning in the process, and see where it takes you.

THE JOY CHOICE IS YOUR CHOICE

I created the Joy Choice to help those of us who can't count on automatic habits, who want to resolve the inner conflicts that keep getting in the way, and who want to learn how to better harness our executive functions through the positivity, meaning, and joy that science suggests drive consistent healthy eating and physical activity decisions. Within the Joy Choice, learning lasting change is how we develop the *real* knowledge we need at the moment of choice.[7] It's our new know-*how* for transforming our negative eating and exercise experiences into positive ones, and a tactical way of thinking about our decision making process that lets us stay the course—not only in spite of setbacks, but by learning what they have to teach us along the way.

Learning lasting change isn't about what we do "in theory." Instead, it's about what we do on the ground as we live each day, learning to strategically and playfully navigate our choice points, continuing to build our real knowledge and slicing and dicing skills as we go. It doesn't matter if the choice point is about not feeling motivated, wanting to be with our kids, eating something special at a celebration, having less time than our original plan needed, or something else. What does matter is that we are prepared to assess our choice points, harnessing our power to self-observe and think strategically so we can learn how to pivot when needed.

The Joy Choice is *your* choice. It is always the option that resonates with both your deepest self-knowledge and with your real-life needs. When you pick the Joy Choice, you create consistency, not perfection. It is a type of wayfinding in which you continually, thoughtfully orient yourself with curiosity to the various choices and tradeoffs on your path *in this moment* so you can effectively make your way from choice to choice, experience to experience, *always* learning lasting change as you go.

EPILOGUE
THE EVER-CHANGING SWEET SPOT OF LASTING CHANGE

I BEGAN THIS BOOK ASKING YOU TO FORGET ABOUT AIMING FOR SUSTAINABLE behavior change and put your full attention on the in-the-moment challenges your eating and exercise plans constantly face. "Sustainable behavior change" implies the ultimate goal: a behavior changed forever. But this framing ignores the busy context that surrounds that goal. In a world that is constantly moving forward, that aspiration can distract us from a more strategic focus: on what is right in front of us, at *this* moment.

When we put our attention at the choice point—the point of conflict between our well-crafted eating or exercise plan and the messy, real-life circumstances that challenge it—we see a very different picture. This gives us a new opportunity: to make a choice *right now* that keeps us moving forward, creating the consistency we've always hoped to achieve. While these ideas might appear overly simple, research suggests that they are sufficiently powerful to drive changes that last.

At each choice point, we are ready to pull out the POP! decision tool, helping us create our new story of lasting behavior change.

First the *fun* part, we POP our plan! Then, we move on to the three steps:

We PAUSE to focus our attention on the moment, filtering out our old reactive responses, acknowledging them, and then stepping over the TRAPs that used to disrupt our decisions. This pause lets us engage our thinking, especially our mental flexibility, allowing us to open the rigid gates of *shoulds* and step into the flow of possibilities.

Now we are ready to OPEN OUR OPTIONS AND PLAY, curious about what else is possible and identifying workarounds that will let us do at least part of our original plan. We've already redefined success as doing something rather than nothing. Now we are in *ever play* mode, freed up to see choice points as genuine opportunities to choose through curiosity, purpose, and play.

Finally, we're ready to PICK the option that works best *now*, in *this* moment, with *these* variables, allowing it to be the perfect *imperfect* option that satisfies our unique combination of needs. Our choice is *our* choice. It no longer represents overcoming perceived deficiencies, following someone else's rules, or being selfish. We make room for the unanticipated while still meeting our own self-care needs, simultaneously renewing our energetic resources for the people, goals, and projects we care most about.

And that's our JOY CHOICE! We've reframed the purpose and meaning of healthy eating and exercise in ways that significantly increase their true value to us. As we reflect on the Joy Choice we just picked, however small, we know that it delivers resources both to ourselves and to our day. We recognize this high-value outcome and carry that wisdom forward with us as our new driver, supporting our executive functions, and helping make future decisions even more effortless.

WE'RE ALL DIFFERENT AND NEED DIFFERENT THINGS. MY HOPE is that you have fun playing with these ideas and possibilities in your own life and in the process discover what resonates and works best for you. The power of truly feeling in charge of your own eating and exercise choices cannot be overstated. This includes just *knowing* that in being self-determined you are better supporting your executive functioning team: working memory, flexible thinking, and inhibition. It doesn't matter what our innate executive functioning abilities are to benefit from the Joy Choice and POP! What does matter is that we proactively take the opportunities to choose that present themselves because they allow us to continue making the small daily decisions that keep us in sync with ourselves and the people and things that matter most.

Welcome to the Joy Choice, the ever-changing sweet spot of lasting change in eating and exercise.

APPENDIX A

Getting Started Picking the Joy Choice:
An Eating Example

A FEW YEARS AGO, ON A FLIGHT TO NEW YORK CITY, MY SEATMATE AND I introduced ourselves and fell into conversation about our lives. Kara told me she had her own small business and that she was engaged to be married to a great guy. In preparation for their wedding the following year, they decided to get "super healthy" to start their life together off right.

"That's awesome," I said, and began to tell her about my career focus on creating sustainable self-care behaviors. Kara excitedly cut me off, diving into the details of their new healthy living project. Their plan was ambitious! They had decided to wake up Monday through Friday at four a.m. to be more productive, meditate for twenty minutes every night before bed, exercise for forty-five to sixty minutes every day, and eat better. After she finished her litany of pro-health plans, she paused to ask my opinion about their endeavor.

I gathered my thoughts before responding. I wanted to be honest, but I also didn't want to say anything that might burst her couple bubble. So, I told Kara about a policy that guides my work with every client. "We get a lot messages from friends, family, and the media about how to be healthy and take good care of ourselves, and the benefits of doing it all. The focus is always on improving our health *now*, changing our behavior *now*, feeling better *now* from meditating, exercising, getting enough sleep, eating better, and on and on! So, naturally, we want to have all of these wonderful benefits and we jump in with both feet determined to change it all *now*."

"Right!" she said, nodding. "So, what's the problem?"

"Well, let me ask you a question. Do you care about achieving lasting change in those healthy behaviors or just about the idea of starting off your life together doing them?"

"I don't know," she said. "Is there a difference?"

"Well, there are generally different strategies for adopting life-style behaviors if our ultimate goal is lasting change, versus just being focused on starting and 'getting to it.' Our societal behavior change narrative encourages us to jump in and change everything, just like you're talking about doing. But it has *not* taught us to start a change in behavior in ways that can really last."

She told me that they hadn't really talked about what comes after the wedding. "That's typical," I said. "Most people don't think beyond their focal, motivating goal. But when I work with clients on creating lasting changes, I ask them to focus on a *single* behavior at a time. My perspective is this: If we aim to sustain a behavior, it has to be integrated into our lives in realistic ways that can ride the waves of life's ups and downs. When we focus on just one behavior to start, we learn a lot about how to do it, and then we can more easily add the next behavior." Kara was nodding in agreement, so I continued.

"To adopt a behavior into our lives in ways we can sustain—that can actually fit into the reality of our hectic lives—we need to learn lasting change *with that behavior*. We need to learn the things that tend to derail it, the solutions that work or don't work, and the choices we make that help us keep it going. And out of those insights and experiences, we gain a mastery of navigating the challenges that our desired behavior faces every day.

"Every plan or intended decision faces its own 'choice points,' the moments it get challenged," I explained. "Whether it's eating or exercise or meditating or sleeping or anything else, it's nearly impossible to put this level of attention on more than one complex behavior at a time. I ask my clients to focus on successfully steering a course through these choice points—these never-ending opportunities to choose when we are challenged by unexpected events or needs in our real lives. It might only be one behavior, but ultimately that behavior is made up of thousands upon thousands of decisions over a lifetime. Our goal is to understand how we can make those decisions more effortlessly, in ways that meet our whole range of needs and keep us successfully moving forward."

At that moment, the plane began its descent. We'd be landing in a few minutes.

I could see that Kara was taking it all in, and was clearly perplexed. "It's not as hard as you think," I said, smiling. "If we had more time I could explain, but there is an easy decision-making technique we can use at these choice points to us guide forward, past the challenges." As the wheels hit the runway, I suggested she speak with her fiancé about these ideas so they could decide together what they were really after with their project. We exchanged contact info and said our good-byes.

About a month later, Kara reached out to me and informed me that she and her fiancé had decided to expand their goal from just targeting their nuptials to cultivating lasting change. They also agreed that focusing on changing only one new behavior at a time made a lot of sense—especially while planning a wedding at the same time! Her fiancé, she said, had chosen to focus on daily meditation. Kara, however, felt that improving her eating practices would be most helpful and asked if I would work with her.

Read on to see how we got started, and how you can get started too.

KARA GETS STARTED WITH THE JOY CHOICE

Kara's story is a great setup for thinking about how you, too, can get started using the Joy Choice in your own life. Whether you already have a specific eating or exercise plan in play, or want to identify one, getting started begins with picking one specific behavior that you want to target for lasting change. "Kara, using the POP! decision tool is how you learn to successfully navigate choices points, so that's what we need to focus on now," I explained.

PRE-POP! MAKE A PLAN THAT TARGETS ONE NEW BEHAVIOR

Kara told me she wanted to make changes in eating because she tended to skip meals and knew that it dragged down her energy level throughout the day. She also ended up feeling really hungry at night and overeating, which sometimes gave her heartburn and actually made it hard for her to get to sleep. She felt pretty motivated to stop skipping meals, she just wasn't sure how to start.

"It's a lot easier for my fiancé to learn to meditate every morning than it is for me to get a handle on my eating," said Kara. "All he has to do is wake up and sit down."

"You're not wrong about meditation having fewer components as a target behavior," I agreed. "Changing our eating behavior is generally more complex than meditating every morning or even changing the amount we're physically active. It's not that those behaviors take no effort; exercise and meditation just don't have the same logistical footprint and number of choice points across our full day. So, it's helpful to acknowledge this when you are getting ready to change your eating behavior!"

I explained that the complexity involved with food and eating is truly impressive. "There can be layers of prep—meal planning, shopping, cooking, family food preferences, mealtimes. In addition, there's an abundance of food everywhere—at work, at social gatherings, at restaurants, in the grocery store itself—which can make it challenging to stick with our food plans. Add to this the variables related to hunger, fullness, stress, and the social and emotional functions food serves, from comfort to reward to celebration..."

"No wonder I've had so many challenges related to eating," said Kara.

"That's why we need to simplify, even within eating," I said. "Many people try to make a boatload of eating-related changes at the same time—no snacking, stay away from sugar, eat more fruits and veggies, eat only whole foods, eat dinner before six p.m., and more! But as you can likely see, that strategy is actually very similar to starting several different behaviors at the same time. Even though all the changes relate to eating, having so many to pay attention to doesn't let us focus on a *specific* target we can learn the ins and outs of. This is a tactical issue that needs tactical thinking."

"Let's start by formally defining one *specific* change in eating to focus on. Consider this your target behavior." I asked her to take an observer perspective on her eating and look at *which* aspect of eating she thought would be most beneficial to change at that time. As she thought about it, she realized that being vague about "improving her eating" was what was getting her in trouble.

"I think what would be most helpful would be to sit at the table—any table, because realistically I won't always be at my own kitchen table!—and eat three real meals a day, consisting of foods I will feel good about eating. Plus," she smiled, "that also means I have to take a break from work and not just cram an energy bar in my mouth."

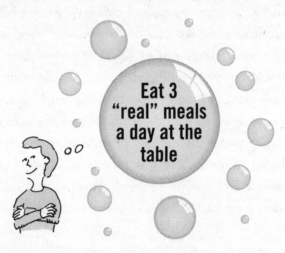

Popping our original plan immediately shifts us into solution mode. By its very nature, the POP! decision tool springs us into action to help us think on our feet, letting us successfully navigate our choice points whenever they arise. That doesn't mean that POP! won't benefit from a little prep, either, especially when it comes to eating-related goals like Kara's.

PRE-POP! MEMORIZE THE "POP!" STEPS

I explained that the acronym POP stands for the three-step sequence that you use at choice points: Pause, Open up your options and play, and Pick the Joy Choice. As an acronym, it is specifically designed to be easy to remember so you can quickly retrieve the POP steps from your long-term memory. "Makes sense," said Kara. "Any tips?"

"One way to get POP! into your long-term memory is to use repetition," I replied. "You can say over and over, 'POP! Pause, Open up your options and play, and Pick the Joy Choice.' Then, try to recall the three steps throughout the day until you have memorized POP!" Kara thought that was hilarious. "It sounds easy, but I'm not sure I'll remember what they all stand for..."

"Another idea is to write it on sticky notes," I said. "Put them up in a few places in your house and where you work, read them throughout the day, and try to say them, without looking. Or if you need a memory aid that you can call up when needed, create a contact in your phone called 'POP!' and write out the three POP! steps in the notes so you can easily access it."

If you're at the same Pre-POP! phase as Kara, get familiar with the POP! graphics in *The Joy Choice*. These images were designed for a science-based reason: reviewing them should also help you get the three POP! steps into your long-term memory, ready and waiting for you to retrieve them when needed. Look at them as much as you need to help make this happen.

PRE-POP! LEAN INTO ALTERNATIVES

I told Kara that even though the POP! sequence asks us to open up our options and look for workarounds at choice points that we may not have thought of, it can be helpful to consider possible options before we need them. "Like backup plans, you mean?" Kara asked.

"Yes, there are science-based strategies like 'if-then' plans that can help us prepare a type of backup plan," I said, "but it's important to consider that having a specific backup plan also has the potential to limit your thinking in the moment a conflict arises. By definition, choice points are unexpected, so your if-then plan may not actually be workable in that moment. The point is, you don't want to assume it's a sure thing and be overly committed to it. You just need to be aware of this potential downside so it doesn't take you by surprise and limit your options.

"It can help to just keep your planning simple," I emphasized. "Another preparatory strategy is to try to memorize the three questions that have the potential to help you devise new options: What else? How much? When? But if you have trouble remembering them, then definitely create a phone contact for POP! as a memory aid. And remember that looking at the pictures like the one below can help!"

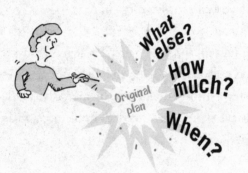

PRE-POP! REMEMBER THE PERFECT *IMPERFECT* OPTION

"That seems like a lot, so I'm going to create that POP! contact right after our session is over," said Kara. "But I'm excited."

"It's actually pretty simple," I said, "and my experience with other clients tells me that it doesn't take long to get into using POP! and have fun with it. But if you're really stuck, just remember this one basic thing: The very best way to prep to POP! isn't a technique at all. It is simply *believing* that there is almost always at least one perfect *imperfect* option. This will automatically get you out of either-or thinking so you can start playing with the possibilities."

But Kara didn't have the luxury of doing much prep because her first choice point happened the day after our initial session.

≥POP!≤ KARA LEARNS TO POP!

It was the last day to submit taxes to her accountant, due by five p.m., and Kara had been rushing the last two days to finish. But the morning they were due, she found the last part was taking longer than she had anticipated and she needed every minute to reach that deadline.

Her eating plan included a thirty-minute sit-down lunch, which consisted of cooking a grilled cheese sandwich, making a salad, and eating an apple. But when her lunch alarm went off, she looked at the piles of papers on her desk and realized that her planned lunch scenario just couldn't work. She had arrived at her first *choice point*!

LIFE IS HAPPENING, CONFLICTS ARISE...

It's a choice point!

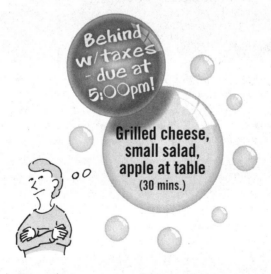

She was bummed—the first day, and already her plans were dashed! But she remembered that to move past this choice point, she had to POP! her original eating plan. She opened up her new POP! contact in her phone and thought to herself, Remember the perfect *imperfect*, and began by POP!ing her plan.

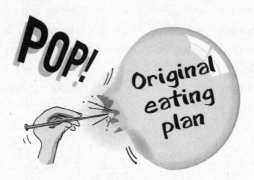

Pause
Open up your options and play
Pick the Joy Choice

1. Pause

Kara *Paused*, and put herself in observer mode.

PAUSE

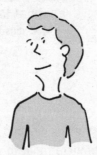

First, she noticed she felt stressed. The only TRAP she iden-
tified was her typical Temptation to just skip lunch. Harnessing that mindfulness, she said out loud, "Kara, let's give this a
try instead. You just started coaching! What are other possible
options instead of your original plans? What trade-offs can you
make?"

2. Open up your options and play

She let herself get into *playful* thinking and *Opened up her
options*. Kara first realized she could grab some cheese and
an apple and quickly eat at her desk, or she could grab the bag
of trail mix in the pantry and graze on it for the rest of the day

OPEN UP YOUR OPTIONS AND PLAY

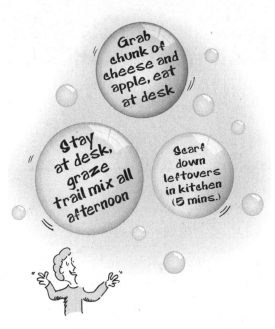

at her desk. But those options, while meeting the perfect *imperfect* criteria, would keep her at her desk all day, something she really wanted to change.

Then, she remembered the leftovers from dinner the night before, and recognized that she could take five or ten minutes to sit down and eat those in the kitchen. This would be quick, it would get her away from her office, respect her plan to sit and eat, and it would give her the energy she needed to finish her tax prep in time. She smiled. But as she was opening the containers, she realized she didn't have the luxury to sit down and eat after all and needed to just scarf down her lunch.

3. Pick the Joy Choice

Kara *Picked this as the Joy Choice* and got the food out of the refrigerator, and quickly ate the leftovers standing up by the kitchen counter.

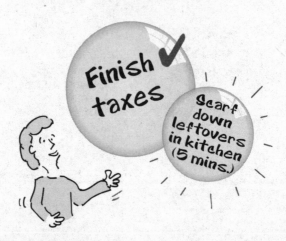

By definition, Kara's Joy Choice was not perfect, but she picked it and owned it, reinforcing the value of doing something instead of nothing and still meeting her five p.m. tax deadline.

POST-POP! REFLECTING ON WHAT HAPPENED

At our next session I asked Kara how she had felt from picking that Joy Choice. "I know it was not the optimal choice," she said, "but I was still excited because I actually did it!" Her baseline had been skipping lunch and feeling depleted. That afternoon, she noticed that she had more energy and was thinking more clearly. "It wasn't as hard as I thought it would be to come up with alternatives," Kara said. "I was proud of myself and super pleased with the results. I was skeptical at first, but it was actually fun to do."

Conscious thinking engages our executive functions and lets us POP! But we shift from *using* the POP! tool to *learning lasting change* when we take an observer's perspective on each POP!, reflecting back on how it went, the benefits it delivered to our day, what worked, what didn't, what we might want to try next time. Aligned with research,[1] I've found that when clients review their past strategies and outcomes in this metacognitive way, it cultivates curiosity and creativity and fosters the real knowledge and confidence that underlies perseverance.

As Kara discovered, by its very nature any Joy Choice is a HUGE WIN. But that doesn't mean we can't get better at POP!ing our plan and using the POP! decision tool. Thinking in this way is new for many, and sometimes it takes time to learn to get into the playful and positive mindset that expands our thinking and solution finding. But I encourage you to stay with it and keep learning about yourself, your options, your possibilities.

Observing ourselves like this is what helps us learn the *actual nuts and bolts of* creating an effective and consistent decision-making process. When we ask questions like *What didn't work well the last time?* and *What can I improve to get the results I want next time?* it gives us the awareness we need to keep getting better on our journey of learning lasting change.

Science shows that *how* we show up for ourselves in the face of setbacks matters. In the old behavior change story, we labeled ourselves as incompetent or failures when things didn't work out as planned. This type of self-assessment and thinking doesn't only *feel* demotivating, science shows it actually is! Metacognition lets us notice when we engage in this counterproductive self-talk. In any worthy learning process, there is no place for negative self-judgments or self-recrimination when we experience bumps in the road. Instead, we can learn to assess our choice point outcomes with self-compassion, which research finds better (*much* better!) facilitates resilience and perseverance toward the lasting change we're after.[2]

USE YOUR RESOURCES, AND SOME OF MINE

You don't need to have a coach to learn lasting change. You don't have to be brilliant or have a will of steel either. The Joy Choice process was designed for *everyone* to lean on. Here are a few inner and outer resources you can use.

Include your family in the Joy Choice.

The beauty of the Joy Choice is that it enables your choices to serve not only your exercise or eating needs, but the changing needs of those you care about most. So, why not invite these others to join you?

You don't have to go it alone; you can bring your whole family into Joy Choice thinking! When it comes to our behavior change projects, having our whole family in on the conversation helps create a supportive and even enjoyable structure. Bringing our kids on board with conversations about learning lasting change is important. It helps *them* develop wise insights about their choices and cultivate positive relationships with healthy eating and exercise that have the potential to last a lifetime, and reinforces *you* in picking the Joy Choice.

Two great children's books to help your children learn adaptive thinking about healthy eating and physical activity are *The Rechargeables: Eat Move Sleep* by Tom Rath[3] and *How to Raise a Mindful Eater: 8 Powerful Principles for Transforming Your Child's Relationship with Food* by Maryann Jacobsen.[4]

Share the Joy Choice with friends, colleagues, and your community.

Your friends, community, and colleagues can also support this journey and become scaffolding around the Joy Choice. Having a supportive and enthusiastic context for your behavior change projects helps more than I could ever say. And it should help them too!

In work I've done helping organizations shift the cultural mindset, we've created social media and other types of programs promoting these new insights to inspire employees to think about and discuss these new ideas with one another and as an organization. This helps foster the important social metacognition that helps contribute to culture change.

If you are in a book club, reading *The Joy Choice* is a great way to start talking about and spreading these ideas. You'll find a discussion guide with provocative discussion-generating questions on my website[5] for this purpose.

Make sure your greater goals for better eating and exercise are truly yours.

Our greater goals for changing our eating and exercise behaviors *matter*: They deeply influence the emotional tone of the relationship we have with these behaviors. Initiating changes out of *shoulds*, shame, or other negative feelings triggers the decision disruptors that TRAP our thinking and pull us under at choice points, derailing our desired decision making.

Don't worry if you don't know what your relationship with food is; you can start from wherever you are. Just remember to maintain the high-level (metacognitive) "observer" perspective we talked about. That way, you can notice if and when you find yourself feeling rebellious, just "meh," stuck in Perfection, or whatever. If so, those are hints that you might benefit from doing more focused work on your *relationship with* eating (or exercise if that is your current focus) before you work on trying to incorporate and integrate changes into your life. If your relationship with your desired change feels negative, this will prevent you from learning lasting change. But there are resources and professionals who can help with this.

As a first step, to work on creating a more positive relationship with eating, you can read about more mindful, intuitive eating in the go-to text by Evelyn Tribole and Elyse Resch, *Intuitive Eating*.[6] When I first learned to appreciate the wisdom of the intuitive eating approach, it was long before it became the respected and mainstream approach it is now, helping people escape the vicious cycle caused by "dieting" and learn to eat in more mindful, healthier, and positive ways.

I wrote my first book, *No Sweat*,[7] for individuals struggling with exercise and physical activity because it feels negative or like a "should." If this is your issue, you can easily transform exercise from feeling like a chore into a gift by following the scientifically supported method described in the book. Research in real-world contexts suggests this method produces long-term change, and I continue to get emails from people sharing their exciting stories of transformation with me. *No Sweat* has become a core text to train professionals in health coaching and health counseling within university curricula and certification programs.

Get skilled at opening up, flexible thinking, and creating new possibilities.

Getting out of the Perfection mindset, leaning into the unknown, being open and playful, and even celebrating the failure of our original plan is a critical part of learning to make the Joy Choice consistently, keeping you on the path of lasting change. While my recommendations for this area might seem strange in the context of a book on healthy eating and exercise, they are very much on topic. The first one is an inspiring parenting book by Daniel Siegel and Tina Payne Bryson, *The Yes Brain: How to Cultivate Courage, Curiosity, and Resilience in Your Child*.[8] This brain-based book offers integrative and easy to use science- and practice-based insights that shed light on how to cultivate a mindful receptivity, resilience, and well-being in our children that I believe can help everyone learn to do this, including us grown-ups. The second book, *Getting to Yes with Yourself: How to Get What You Truly Want*, by renowned negotiation expert William Ury,[9] explains that our natural tendency to think in all-or-nothing, win-lose ways is the greatest obstacle to successful negotiations. Ury teaches how we can get to yes with ourselves through increased self-awareness and reframing as key parts of creating the cycle of winning we're after.

Until I wrote this section, I didn't even realize that both titles I was recommending have "yes" in them! This made me chuckle. It also hit home that being open and receptive rather than reactive and closed is the mental perspective for resilient decision making *across life arenas*—from helping our kids develop resilience and well-being to opening ourselves up through a mindset that gets us the win-win-win to staying the course with healthy eating and exercise. Regardless of what we're aiming for, curiosity, self-awareness, self-compassion, strategic framing, flexibility, and compromise are key ingredients for success.

There will always be differences between the strategies and approaches that work for people. But something that is not different: *we all need* the self-awareness and ability to reflect on and observe our own thoughts, beliefs, experiences, and outcomes to identify which programs, tools, and strategies will best work for each of us. We are each a unique human being, so let's honor that fact by honoring ourselves as we navigate our unique path of lasting change.

APPENDIX B

Professional Goals and Industry Cases

I WROTE *THE JOY CHOICE* NOT ONLY FOR INDIVIDUALS, BUT ALSO WITH YOU and your professional challenges and goals in mind. I especially wanted to explain the new science and give you new, easy-to-use concepts for the meaningful work you do with patients, clients, employees, and consumers. The underlying principles are being used in counseling individuals, and they are also being used to guide the design of next-generation behavior change solutions across contexts.

A NOTE TO PROFESSIONALS

If you are a professional who works within health care, organizational well-being, fitness, or health coaching, you have firsthand experience with the old behavior change story, and the knowledge that this approach does not work for the vast majority. Changing the way we think and do things is never easy; but when these changes engender positivity and purpose, they can be much easier for everyone—including professionals and organizations—to adopt.

One of the key tenets of *The Joy Choice* is that flexibility equals feasibility. As stories in the book showed, people are often challenged to accept this concept because it somehow feels like it's "dumbing down" what they should "really" be doing. As you've seen, that isn't the case! A key part of your challenge is to help people understand the true opportunity for the well-being and sustainability that picking the Joy Choice can bring them. Choosing to do *something*—even if it isn't ideal—is almost always better than defaulting to the all-or-nothing mindset, which often leads us to just give up altogether. Choosing the perfect *imperfect* option is choosing the *something* that cultivates consistency, the behavioral resilience that *is* lasting change.

Many books on behavior change tend to group eating and exercise together with other types of behavioral changes; but these two behaviors are different from other behaviors in important respects. Like other self-care behaviors, healthy eating and regular exercise are both wonderful ways to take care of ourselves. Yet unlike other behaviors, they have unfortunately been contaminated for many by a cultural narrative that creates stigma and shame, which in turn engenders negative beliefs and experiences associated with them. Naming and discussing the four core decision TRAPs—Temptation, Rebellion, Accommodation, and Perfection—is a way to call out these negative forces, reducing their power over our attention at choice points. In general, these damaging issues constitute literal forces that easily disrupt adaptive thinking at choice points. So, taking these issues seriously and helping people understand them is an important part of the science-based Joy Choice solution.

Many traditional behavior change programs have tended to arrive wrapped up in seriousness and high stakes. The Joy Choice puts a new frame around eating and exercise choice points, transforming them from moments of stress to opportunities to be creative and play and learn more about ourselves. In conjunction with my goal of helping people create lasting change in these behaviors, I developed these ideas and tools to make the whole process *fun*—for individuals, for you in your work, and even for me! This work is my calling, and I have a blast doing it.

The Joy Choice solution is constructed from easy-to-understand components:

+ the perfect *imperfect* option that helps build consistency;
+ the three strategies to support our executive functioning: Simplify, Play, and Choose Joy; and
+ the POP! decision tool, which embodies these three strategies, is easy to recall at choice points, and efficiently guides us to picking the Joy Choice!

These components are easily taught and purposely designed to be memorable and compelling. They can be brought up via coaching and counseling discussions, and employed in other ways (such as book club discussions, social media–based programming, and self-care campaigns) to help you help your end users rethink eating and exercise decision making so you can achieve your mutual long-term goals.

Let's look at a few examples of how aligned principles are being operationalized and scaled within the fitness, corporate well-being, and health-care industries.

FITNESS INDUSTRY: EXPERIENCE AND COMMUNITY MATTERS

Health, wellness, and fitness industries have already started to adopt practices that the new science suggests will bring more positive and lasting results. They are doing this by taking into account not only the individual's health but the whole person, including their pleasure, preferences, and life context. Interestingly, the COVID-19 pandemic brought the fitness industry—gyms, equipment companies, personal trainers—to an epiphany. They've known for decades that the usual approach to "fitness" and exercise has attracted only a limited population and intimidated many others. Industry leaders are now beginning to think more intentionally about how they can create a new meaning for exercise to connect with those who are actually made uncomfortable by the very idea of fitness and exercise.

When I spoke about this to Brent Darden, past president and CEO of IHRSA–The Global Health & Fitness Association, he told me that "To a degree, the health and fitness industry has been its own worst enemy. Shifting the narrative from a focus on aesthetics, weight loss, and 'fitness' toward general well-being is a trend in the right direction."[1] The fitness industry is starting to learn how to shift this conversation away from these traditional (and tired) outcomes toward new ones, helping gym members and personal training clients discover more deeply compelling reasons for consistent exercise and healthy eating, experiences that also deliver more positive feelings and better results.

To help me understand more about this industry shift on the ground, I interviewed Sara Hodson, president and CEO of LIVE WELL Exercise Clinic, a fast-growing fitness franchise in Canada, and president of the Fitness Industry Council of Canada. She had a lot to say about how her company addresses this issue: "Most of our members come to us to have a conversation about losing weight," she said. "But we're ready and waiting to tackle that. Through our onboarding process we ask a series of questions aimed at helping them shift from thinking about losing weight to thinking about how they can live their life to the fullest. The numbers on the scale always let us down and we quit the things that let us down. We take the focus away from the scale and help them uncover the deeper values and their real *why* for being here, and ask them to start creating more positive experiences through their choices. They tell us they are surprisingly relieved that their work with us isn't about harsh diets and strenuous exercise. After we implemented this system, our one-year retention increased from 38 percent to 71 percent."[2]

Sara's further comments about the fitness industry post-pandemic align with my experience: that people have never thought about their health in the way they do today. The fitness industry is at a true crossroads. People want physical activity to help address their physical, mental, *and* social health. Sara said that "fitness facilities and gyms, even more so after COVID, are creating community and culture around creating meaningful change. We're going way beyond the body's fitness level to our deepest wish—to connect with others." The idea that engaging in physical activity can become a wonderful vehicle of connection and community aligns with research showing that *connection*, as a value and experience, is highly motivating on a deep human level and a physically active one too.[3]

But these exciting new community-building initiatives are going beyond just cultivating connections between people. Businesses are cropping up to forge new interorganizational partnerships, helping health and fitness clubs transform from being "just a gym people exercise in" into an "essential community resource" that helps improve the health of the whole community. Amy Bantham, DrPH, CEO and founder of Move to Live More, told me about her work forming collaborations between fitness and health clubs and community stakeholders, such as local clinics and schools. "Using data and even anecdotes, we can discover how isolated and inactive kids in a community have become. Then, together, the club and school district might realize the need for a physical activity program that can address the most pressing mental and physical health needs of the students. If we learn that the school lacks the people and infrastructure to execute the program, the club can step up with certified youth fitness specialists and the physical space or technology to run the program virtually or in person."[4] This new vision frames physical activity and health as essentially intertwined (as of course they are) and in need of being interconnected across the different spaces within which we live our lives. Similar to the Joy Choice, this holistic initiative assumes that healthy behavior initiatives will be more successful when they are integrated across our many life contexts.

ORGANIZATIONAL WELL-BEING: SUPPORTING EMPLOYEE WELL-BEING IN NEW WAYS

Given that so many people have trouble sticking with their eating and exercise goals, it is perhaps not surprising that organizations attempting to boost their employees' health have experienced challenges with program adherence. Urged on by these failures, the corporate wellness arena has been interested in finding out what they need to do differently. Out of this self-reflection has come the recognition that past strategies, where employers create the rules, don't work long-term.

These industries are now intentionally trying to learn lasting change strategies, including using science-based communication principles, reframing their "health" messages to employees, and even changing internal department names to emphasize the whole person. LuAnn Heinen, vice president of Business Group on Health, affirmed that "Employers have been changing their approach. We've learned that top-down strategies don't work and that employees need to have autonomy over how they take better care of themselves. In our industry, there is a growing trend to give employees opportunities to define their own health-related needs, wants, and priorities and provide the right programming to help them achieve those things."[5]

Heinen's insight dovetails nicely with what Laura Putnam, CEO of Motion Infusion and author of *Workplace Wellness That Works*, told me about how some organizations are implementing these ideas. "Feeling autonomous over our own well-being is critical—as in, having the autonomy to choose what well-being means to us and how we go about achieving it. The question then becomes: Do we have the freedom to actually pursue it? Within the context of where we work, managers wield a surprising level of influence. Each manager is uniquely positioned to either facilitate or unwittingly undermine their team members' engagement with well-being. Therefore, when managers take explicit measures to give permission and create the conditions, individual employees are more likely to feel enabled to pursue their version of well-being especially at work."[6]

This is exactly the kind of approach that Blue Cross Blue Shield of North Dakota (BCBSND) is taking toward well-being. In 2020, when CEO and president Daniel Conrad took the helm of BCBSND, he arrived with a mission to make the well-being of employees a top company priority. The intent was to give each employee a choice in deciding what well-being looks like for them, while making sure that the larger culture supports that. This call for a cultural shift was needed to ensure that well-being would go beyond being a platitude to becoming fully integrated into the day-to-day of business. With the explicit directive from Conrad, over the past year and a half BCBSND has been addressing the organizational forces that inform behaviors: empowering managers to promote well-being within their teams, fostering an "all-in" cooperation across all departments, adding company-wide practices that normalize self-care, and making well-being more holistic, meaningful, and inclusive. As evidenced by the data, these efforts are making a difference. Over the period of 2020 to 2021, 81 percent of employees report feeling that BCBSND cares about their well-being (up significantly from 64 percent in 2020). Perhaps most remarkably, employees and managers are reporting an *increase* in overall well-being (up 24 percent for employees and up 36 percent for managers from 2020 to 2021), even in the midst of the pandemic.[7]

In contrast to the liabilities associated with the sleepless leaders in the research discussed in the Accommodation chapter, the intentional decision of BCBSND's top leaders to create policies cultivating a culture of self-care and well-being is clearly paying dividends.

HEALTH CARE: TAILORING TREATMENT TO EACH PATIENT'S NEEDS

Organizations within health care are also learning lasting change, and the emphasis on patient-centered care continues to grow. This means providing care that is respectful of and responsive to the patient as an *individual*, ensuring that the care and clinical decisions for each person is tailored to their unique needs.[8] Research shows that having clinicians and patients "cocreate" treatment and care in this way benefits patient satisfaction in addition to their physical and social well-being.[9]

The Mayo Clinic's "minimally disruptive medicine" (MDM) is a model of care that does this well. It starts by working with the patient to understand what their situation calls for and then to figure out what treatment plan makes the most sense. This type of tailored, collaborative approach by which patients and clinicians cocreate a treatment plan is sometimes called shared decision making.[10] MDM's objective is to achieve the goals of each patient while also reducing the treatment burden and patient overwhelm. Dr. Victor Montori, the codeveloper of MDM and professor of medicine at Mayo Clinic, told me: "Our old practice in medicine had been to ask patients to do *more* through their prescribed treatment, even when they did not have the capacity to do more because they are busy being a parent, a spouse, a worker, or a volunteer. With MDM, we acknowledge these challenges and collaborate with them to figure out the treatment plan. And even if the plan doesn't work, we've developed a relationship that lets us apply what we learned to try something else that might."[11] I am so heartened by the flexibility deployed approach to health care that treats patients through taking the context of their full set of needs into account, which is *the exact opposite* of the traditional "prescription constriction" approach that was discussed in the chapter on Play.

Another example of an approach to tailor care to the individual patient relates to prescribing physical activity. In this regard, I developed a tool called "Choose to M.O.V.E.: Move to Optimize Vitality and Enjoyment," depicted in the figure. This tool is used to train clinicians how to tailor physical activity counseling to each patient, emphasizing how to help patients learn to create the positive experiences through movement that predict ongoing participation. In contrast to the typical "prescription pad" approach that guides clinicians to prescribe a "dose" of physical activity (e.g., intensity level, duration) to patients, Choose to M.O.V.E. changes the frame from dose-based, doctor-prescribed to patient-centered and experience-focused. It invites patients to consider what type(s) of *positive experiences* they want to have from being active, and to select the physical activities that will deliver these positive experiences, framing this as a process of learning.[12]

Cindy Lin, MD, clinical associate professor of Sports & Spine Medicine and associate director of Clinical Innovation at The Sports Institute at University of Washington Medical Center, explains that "the Choose to M.O.V.E. prescription helps me engage my patients in making a plan to get active. I typically use it at the end of a clinic visit

Choose to **M.O.V.E.**!

Move to **O**ptimize your **V**itality and **E**njoyment!

NAME:_____ DATE:_____

What positive experiences do you want from being physically active?
(Check your top 2)

☐ **Vitality**   ☐ **Well-being**   ☐ **Connection**
☐ **Less Stress**   ☐ **Better mood**   ☐ **Clear my mind**
☐ **Stronger**   ☐ **Feel in control**   ☐ **Other:** _____
☐ **Relaxed**   ☐ **Enjoyment/fun**   _____
☐ **Joyful**   ☐ **Less anxious**   _____

What type of movement is most likely to bring these experiences
to you?_____
_____
_____

What would a realistic goal be for starting this week?_____
_____
_____

How can I support you in learning how to move more?_____
_____
_____
_____

and they can fill it out while I'm entering orders and referrals so it
doesn't take much time out of the visit. We then scan a copy to their
medical records so we can check in on their progress at the next visit
and they take their own copy home. Along with using the physical

activity vital sign to identify inactive patients, this is a great tool for 'prescribing' activity in patient-centered ways."[13]

THIS IS AN EXCITING TIME OF REFLECTION AND RECKONING regardless of industry, product, service, or profession. Now is the moment to reflect seriously about what hasn't worked and why, and what we as a society can learn from our past experiences and use going forward on this new path of learning lasting change. The examples in this appendix showcase organizations that are working to support the individual's pursuit of well-being. They demonstrate how we can partner with individuals in flexible ways and support decision making through adaptive, science-based strategies—from designing positive experiences to tailoring treatment plans to each unique patient, creating community-based partnerships and autonomy-supportive policies. At their heart, such policies endeavor to meet each person's unique full set of needs and find realistic, perfect *imperfect* solutions rather than take overly perfectionistic, simplistic or one-size-fits-all approaches. I am excited to see these growing trends taking hold, contributing to transforming the behavior change story on a larger scale. Helping professionals and organizations learn how to apply or scale cutting-edge science in their work assisting others to change health-related behaviors in lasting ways is something I'm very passionate about. For more information on my trainings and resources related to using these ideas in your work, please visit MichelleSegar .com.

I wrote this book to help individuals and the professionals and organizations that care about supporting them learn how to create lasting changes in healthier eating and regular physical activity. But with a background also in public health and health care policy, I need to acknowledge that many people do not have the privilege of working on their health behaviors because they are under-resourced and have more extreme concerns related to daily survival. While books can be helpful in many ways and for many people, we need cross-sector partnerships and national policies to improve population-level health and well-being. Yet, I hope that some of the new thinking discussed in *The Joy Choice* might also contribute to the health and well-being of those working hard to implement these important structural-level solutions.

ACKNOWLEDGMENTS

Something that never ceases to astound and delight me is the extent to which ideas and concepts are amplified and enhanced through working with others. Writing *The Joy Choice* has been an incredible journey, full of learning, creativity, humility, and collaboration. Partnering with and being assisted by the many special people below has been among the greatest gifts I've ever received. I am deeply grateful to everyone for their input, guidance, constructive feedback, and inspiration.

It is more than a privilege to work with my developmental editor Naomi Lucks; every part of *The Joy Choice* is so much better because of her ingenuity, authenticity, and humor. Our work together is always very fun and creative. The wonderful Joy Choice graphics also come out of a meaningful partnership I have with the very talented Jeannette Gutierrez and Chris Bidlack.

A heartfelt thank-you goes to my agent, Giles Anderson, who not only believed in this idea at an early stage but also had key insights that shaped its successful direction. I am also very grateful to Hachette Go senior editor Dan Ambrosio for believing in the vision of *The Joy Choice*, supporting its birth, and providing insights that guided the narrative in significant ways. A huge thank-you also goes out to the full Hachette Go team that supported me, and to *The Joy Choice* production and promotion team, including Alison Dalafave, Amber Morris, Zachary Polendo, Michelle Aielli, and Quinn Fariel, among many others.

While the concepts, strategies, and tools in *The Joy Choice* are uniquely mine, they reflect an intensive integration of insights across my research, the research and scholarship of many others, my coaching and industry-related work and interviews, as well as many friends, family, and colleagues who provided input into the ideas and narrative. And I wouldn't have it any other way. The bits, pieces, and parts from these numerous different sources and experiences didn't just coalesce together to help me think in bigger and better ways—they made writing this book a creative and collaborative blast.

In addition to the scholars whom I don't personally know but whose work inspired some of my thinking, I want to express my extreme gratitude to the following people whom I do know and who invested their time and energy, from the inception of this book idea through its preproduction days, to speak or brainstorm with me, read parts or all of *The Joy Choice*, and to answer questions or correct mistakes related to the science, narrative, and industry practices:

The scientists and industry leaders who I learned from, many of whom also suggested resources or provided feedback on my ideas and/ or on the narrative, including Caroline Richardson, Scott Barry Kaufman, Emily Falk, Julie Dirksen, John Ratey, Mark Fendrick, Maryann Jacobsen, LuAnn Heinen, Laura Putnam, Cindy Lin, Victor Montori, Sara Hodson, Brent Darden, Gretchen Spreitzer, Rachael Seidler, Tom Dahlborg, Amy Bantham, Ralf Brand, Paddy

Ekkekakis, Michael Stults-Kolehmainen, Ethan Kross, Kate Olscamp, David Hoke, Emily Wyckoff, and Tanya Berry. An extra-special thank-you goes to Joel Nigg and Alison Miller, who carved out time for many conversations about the ins and outs of executive functioning. I learned a great deal about the research of others, and from fields outside my own, and any potential mistakes in relaying this science are mine and mine alone.

My readers, listeners, and feedback givers include Ilene Segar, Carole Horowitz, Aubrey Lopatin, Jill Weaver, my husband and son, Rachel Thompson, Gabrielle Gruber, Jessica Grossmeier, Margie Yaker, Cesar Valdez, Lori Hollander, Kim Stone, Pam Thompson, Khita Whyatt, Cheri McGowan, Anne McGowan, Blake McGowan, Aviva Simonte, Danielle Wiley, Michael Wiley, Heather Glidden, Ann Lynch, Mary Racelis, Preeti Garg, Sam Gottlieb, and Scott Roberts. And a thank-you goes out to Lauryn Fairchild, Katie Althuis, and Cecelia Schmitt for their help gathering early research for the book.

Whether their (anonymous) stories were included in this book or not, my coaching clients have always been among my greatest teachers. Your challenges and wisdom are among the greatest guides on *my* path of learning lasting change. I am privileged to be able to do this important work with you. It is not only deeply meaningful and purpose-driven, but it also helps me learn more about how to translate the latest research into pragmatic methods and engaging ideas that can help people change their behavior in sustainable ways.

Last but not least, *The Joy Choice* was a family affair! I could not have written this book without the extreme love and patience from my husband and son, and their never-ending support over the months I spent immersed in writing *The Joy Choice*. Thank you to Jeff, my beloved and partner of nineteen years. You are my love, support, and anchor, and an incredible father. Thank you to my son, Eli, my greatest gift. You teach me how to be better every day as a mom, human being, and writer. I am also blessed to have had the support and ear of my family, including my parents, Ilene and Bob Segar (Mom, I owe many improvements in this book to you!), my siblings Steve Segar and Andy Getz, Aviva and Jimmy Simonte, my uncle Bruce Aaron, and my in-laws, Carole Horowitz, Michael Horowitz and Betsy Clubine, and Karen and Rob Greenbaum.

NOTES

CHAPTER 1. IS THE POWER OF HABITS ALL IT'S CRACKED UP TO BE FOR HEALTHY EATING AND EXERCISE?

1. E. T. Berkman, "The Neuroscience of Goals and Behavior Change," *Journal of Consulting and Clinical Psychology* 70, no. 1 (March 2018): 28–44, http://doi.org/10.1037/cpb0000094.

2. W. Wood, "Habit in Personality and Social Psychology," *Personality and Social Psychology Review* 21, no. 4 (2017): 389–403.

L. Carden and W. Wood, "Habit Formation and Change," *Current Opinion in Behavioral Sciences*, 20 (2018): 117–122.

3. W. Wood and D. T. Neal, "A New Look at Habits and the Habit-Goal Interface," *Psychological Review* 114 (2007): 843–863.

4. Charles Duhigg, *The Power of Habit: Why We Do What We Do in Life and Business* (New York: Random House, 2014).

5. Wendy Wood, *Good Habits, Bad Habits: The Science of Making Positive Changes That Stick* (New York: Farrar, Straus and Giroux, 2019), 130.

6. William James, *Habit* (New York: Henry Holt, 1890).

7. The Hamilton Project: Age Distribution of Undergraduate Students, by Type of Institution, accessed January 2, 2020, https://www.hamiltonproject .org/charts/age_distribution_of_undergraduate_students_by_type_of _institution.

Campus Explorer: Married College Students, accessed January 2, 2019, https://www.campusexplorer.com/college-advice-tips/CF0064F6/Married-College-Students/.

8. P. Lally et al., "How Habits Are Formed: Modeling Habit Formation in the Real World," *European Journal of Social Psychology* 40, no. 6 (2010): 998–1009.

9. B. M. Galla and A. L. Duckworth, "More Than Resisting Temptation: Beneficial Habits Mediate the Relationship Between Self-Control and Positive Life Outcomes," *Journal of Personality and Social Psychology* 109 (2015): 508–525.

10. R. Ryan and R. Deci, "Self-Determination Theory and the Facilitation of Intrinsic Motivation, Social Development, and Well-Being," *American Psychologist* 55, no. 1 (2000): 68–78.

S. McLachlan et al., "Shame: A Self-Determination Theory Perspective," *Psychology of Neuroscience and Shame*, in *Psychology of Emotions, Motivations and Actions*, ed. R. G. Jackson (2010): 211–224, https://www.research gate.net/profile/Martin-Hagger/publication/258029062_Shame_A_self -determination_theory_perspective/links/5d9cc472a6fdccfd0e84035e /Shame-A-self-determination-theory-perspective.pdf.

Richard M. Ryan and Edward L. Deci, *Self-Determination Theory: Basic Psychological Needs in Motivation, Development, and Wellness*, 1st ed., (New York: Guilford Press, 2017).

R. M. Ryan, J. N. Donald, and E. L. Bradshaw, "Mindfulness and Motivation: A Process View Using Self-Determination Theory," *Current Directions in Psychological Science* 30, no. 4 (2021): 300–306, http://doi .org/10.1177/09637214211009511.

11. B. D. Rosenberg and J. T. Siegel, "A 50-Year Review of Psychological Reactance Theory: Do Not Read This Article," *Motivation Science* 4, no. 4 (2018): 281–300, https://doi.org/10.1037/mot0000091.

Jack W. Brehm, *A Theory of Psychological Reactance* (Cambridge, MA: Academic Press, 1966).

12. S. E. Iso-Ahola, "Exercise: Why It Is a Challenge for Both the Nonconscious and Conscious Mind," *Review of General Psychology* 17, no. 1 (2013): 93–110.

13. R. Brand and P. Ekkekakis, "Affective–Reflective Theory of Physical Inactivity and Exercise," *German Journal of Exercise and Sport Research* 48 (2018): 48–58, https://doi.org/10.1007/s12662-017-0477-9.

14. W. Wood, L. Tam, and M. G. Witt, "Changing Circumstances, Disrupting Habits," *Journal of Personality and Social Psychology* 88, no. 6 (2005): 918–933, https://doi.org/10.1037/0022-3514.88.6.918.

15. M. S. Hagger, "Habit and Physical Activity: Theoretical Advances, Practical Implications, and Agenda for Future Research," *Psychology of Sport and Exercise* 42 (2019): 118–129.

16. B. Gardner, A. L. Rebar, and P. Lally, "'Habitually Deciding' or 'Habitually Doing'? A Response to Hagger (2019)," *Psychology of Sport and Exercise* 47, 1469-0292 (2020): 101539, https://doi.org/10.1016/j.psychsport.2019.05.008.

L. A. Phillips, "Challenging Assumptions About Habit: A Response to Hagger (2019)," *Psychology of Sport and Exercise* 47 (2020): 101502, https://www.sciencedirect.com/science/article/abs/pii/S146902921930130X?via%3Dihub.

Hagger, "Habit and Physical Activity."

17. Wood, "Habit in Personality and Social Psychology."

18. Daniel Kahneman, *Thinking, Fast and Slow* (New York: Farrar, Straus and Giroux, 2010).

J. A. Bargh and T. L. Chartrand, "The Unbearable Automaticity of Being," *American Psychologist* 54 (1999): 462–479.

19. T. Berkman, "The Neuroscience of Goals and Behavior Change," *Journal of Consulting and Clinical Psychology* 70, no. 1 (March 2018): 28–44, https://doi.org/10.1037/cpb0000094.

20. R. F. Baumeister, E. J. Masicampo, and K. D. Vohs, "Do Conscious Thoughts Cause Behavior?" *Annual Review of Psychology* 62 (2011): 331–361.

21. Thrive Global.com, "10 Microsteps That Have Helped Us Enjoy Healthy Eating," https://thriveglobal.com/stories/healthy-eating-nutrition-tips-favorite-microsteps.

22. J. Updegraff and K. Scout, "Substituting Activities Mediates the Effect of Cognitive Flexibility on Physical Activity: A Daily Diary Study," *Journal of Behavioral Medicine* 40 (2017): 669–674.

A. Joki, J. Makela, and A. Fogelholm, "Permissive Flexibility in Successful Lifelong Weight Management: A Qualitative Study Among Finnish Men and Women," *Appetite* 116 (2017): 157–163.

23. M. S. Hagger, "Habit and Physical Activity: Theoretical Advances, Practical Implications, and Agenda for Future Research," *Psychology of Sport and Exercise* 42 (2019): 118–129.

24. G. Judah, B. Gardner, and R. Aunger, "Forming a Flossing Habit: An Exploratory Study of the Psychological Determinants of Habit Formation," *British Journal of Health Psychology* 18 (2013): 338–353.

CHAPTER 2. CHANGING BEHAVIOR AMID THE CHAOS AND STRESS OF OUR CRAZY-BUSY LIVES

1. Dictionary.com, "Chaos," July 2021, https://www.dictionary.com /browse/chaos.

2. Alison Miller, personal communication, June 17, 2020.

3. A. P. Matheny et al., "Bringing Order Out of Chaos: Psychometric Characteristics of the Confusion, Hubbub, and Order Scale," *Journal of Applied Developmental Psychology* 16, no. 3 (1995): 429–444.

4. Daniel J. Levitin, "Why the Modern World Is Bad for Your Brain," *Guardian*, January 18, 2015, accessed June 9, 2021, https://www.theguardian .com/science/2015/jan/18/modern-world-bad-for-brain-daniel-j-levitin -organized-mind-information-overload.

5. "What Is Executive Function?" Understood.org, accessed June 12, 2021, https://www.understood.org/en/learning-thinking-differences/child -learning-disabilities/executive-functioning-issues/what-is-executive-func tion.

6. Levitin, "Why the Modern World Is Bad for Your Brain."

Jon Hamilton, "Think You're Multitasking? Think Again," *NPR Morning Edition*, October 2, 2008, accessed May 23, 2021, https://www.npr.org/tem plates/story/story.php?storyId=95256794.

7. Levitin, "Why the Modern World Is Bad for Your Brain."

8. J. T. Nigg, "Annual Research Review: On the Relations Among Self-Regulation, Self-Control, Executive Functioning, Effortful Control, Cognitive Control, Impulsivity, Risk-Taking, and Inhibition for Developmental Psychopathology," *Journal of Child Psychology and Psychiatry, and Allied Disciplines* 58, no. 4 (2017): 361–383, https://doi.org/10.1111/jcpp.12675.

W. Hofmann et al., "Working Memory Capacity and Self-Regulatory Behavior: Toward an Individual Differences Perspective on Behavior Determination by Automatic Versus Controlled Processes," *Journal of Personality and Social Psychology* 95, no. 4 (October 2008): 962–977, https://doi .10.1037/a0012705, PMID: 18808271.

9. S. Harris and S. Bray, "Effects of Mental Fatigue on Exercise Decision-Making," *Psychology of Sport and Exercise* 44 (2018): 1–8.

10. P. Sheeran and T. L. Webb, "The Intention-Behavior Gap," *Social and Personality Psychology Compass* (2016), https://doi.org/10.1111/spc3.12265.

11. Joel Nigg, phone interview, April 13, 2021.

12. E. T. Berkman, "The Neuroscience of Goals and Behavior Change," *Consulting Psychology Journal* 70, no. 1 (2018): 28–44, https://doi.org/10.1037 /cpb0000094.

13. E. T. Berkman, "Value-Based Choice: An Integrative, Neuroscience-Informed Model of Health Goals," *Psychology & Health* 33, no. 1 (2018): 40–57, https://doi.org/10.1080/08870446.2017.1316847.

CHAPTER 3. WHY WE DON'T "JUST DO IT"

1. Steven J. Dubner, "Episode 306: How to Launch a Behavior Change Revolution," *Freakonomics* (podcast), https://freakonomics.com/podcast /launch-behavior-change-revolution/.

2. Kurt Lewin, *A Dynamic Theory of Personality* (New York: McGraw Hill, 1935).

3. P. L. Yao, L. Laurencelle, and F. Trudeau, "Former Athletes' Lifestyle and Self-Definition Changes After Retirement from Sports," *Journal of Sport and Health Science* 9, no. 4 (July 2020): 376–383, https://doi.org/10.1016/j .jshs.2018.08.006.

4. K. Lewin, "Defining the 'Field at a Given Time,'" *Psychological Review* 50, no. 3 (1943): 292–310, https://doi.org/10.1037/h0062738.

5. Lewin, *A Dynamic Theory of Personality*.

6. E. K. Papies, L. W. Barsalou, and D. Rusz, "Understanding Desire for Food and Drink: A Grounded-Cognition Approach," *Current Directions in Psychological Science* 29, no. 2 (April 2020): 193–198, https://doi.org/10.1177/0963721420904958.

7. M. A. Stults-Kolehmainen et al., "Motivation States for Physical Activity and Sedentary Behavior: Desire, Urge, Wanting, and Craving," *Frontiers in Psychology* 11 (November 6, 2020): 568390, https://doi.org/10.3389/fpsyg.2020.568390.

R. Brand and P. Ekkekakis, "Affective–Reflective Theory of Physical Inactivity and Exercise Foundations and Preliminary Evidence," *German Journal of Exercise and Sport Research* 48, no. 1 (March 2018): 48–58.

CHAPTER 4. DECISION DISRUPTOR #1: TEMPTATION

1. W. Hofmann, M. Friese, and R. W. Wiers, "Impulsive Versus Reflective Influences on Health Behavior: A Theoretical Framework and Empirical Review," *Health Psychology Review*, Issue 2, Volume 2 (2009): 111–137, https://doi.org/10.1080/17437190802617668.

Daniel Kahneman, *Thinking, Fast and Slow* (New York: Farrar, Straus and Giroux, 2013).

2. D. E. Conroy and T. R. Berry, "Automatic Affective Evaluations of Physical Activity," *Exercise and Sport Sciences Reviews* 45, no. 4 (October 2017): 230–237.

L. Alison Phillips, "Challenging Assumptions About Habit: A Response to Hagger," *Psychology of Sport and Exercise* 47 (2019): 101502, ISSN 1469-0292 (2020), https://doi.org/10.1016/j.psychsport.2019.03.005.

3. E. K. Papies, L. W. Barsalou, and D. Rusz, "Understanding Desire for Food and Drink: A Grounded-Cognition Approach," *Current Directions in Psychological Science* 29, no. 2 (April 2020): 193–198, https://doi.org/10.1177/0963721420904958.

R. Brand and P. Ekkekakis, "Affective–Reflective Theory of Physical Inactivity and Exercise," *German Journal of Exercise and Sport Research* 48 (2018): 48–58, https://doi.org/10.1007/s12662-017-0477-9.

4. Brand and Ekkekakis, "Affective–Reflective Theory."

M. A. Stults-Kolehmainen et al., "Motivation States for Physical Activity and Sedentary Behavior: Desire, Urge, Wanting, and Craving," *Frontiers in Psychology* 11 (2020): 568390, https://doi.org/10.3389/fpsyg.2020.568390.

Papies, Barsalou, and Rusz, "Understanding Desire for Food and Drink."

5. Hofmann, Friese, and Wiers, "Impulsive Versus Reflective Influences on Health Behavior."

J. T. Nigg, "Annual Research Review: On the Relations Among Self-Regulation, Self-Control, Executive Functioning, Effortful Control, Cognitive Control, Impulsivity, Risk-Taking, and Inhibition for Developmental Psychopathology," *Journal of Child Psychology and Psychiatry* 58, no. 4 (April 2017): 361–383, http://doi.org/10.1111/jcpp.12675.

6. Hofmann, Friese, and Wiers, "Impulsive Versus Reflective Influences."

E. Ekkekakis and R. Brand, "Exercise Motivation from a Post-cognitivist Perspective," in *Motivation and Self-Regulation in Sport and Exercise*, eds. Chris Englert and Ian Taylor (Milton Park: Routledge, 2021), 20–40.

F. Strack and R. Deutsch, "Reflective and Impulsive Determinants of Social Behavior," *Personality and Social Psychology Review* 8, no. 3 (2004): 220–247.

7. Joel Nigg, phone interview, April 14, 2021.

8. Brand and Ekkekakis, "Affective–Reflective Theory of Physical Inactivity and Exercise."

9. Ekkekakis and Brand, "Exercise Motivation from a Post-cognitivist Perspective."

10. Papies, Barsalou, and Rusz, "Understanding Desire for Food and Drink."

11. Papies, Barsalou, and Rusz, "Understanding Desire for Food and Drink."

12. M. Keesman et al., "Consumption Simulations Induce Salivation to Food Cues," *PLoS One* 11, no. 11 (November 7, 2016): e0165449, https://doi.org/10.1371/journal.pone.0165449.

13. J. Chen, E. K. Papies, and L. W. Barsalou, "A Core Eating Network and Its Modulations Underlie Diverse Eating Phenomena," *Brain and Cognition* 110 (December 2016): 20–42, https://doi.org/10.1016/j.bandc.2016.04.004.

Papies, Barsalou, and Rusz, "Understanding Desire for Food and Drink."

14. F. Grabenhorst, E. T. Rolls, and A. Bilderbeck, "How Cognition Modulates Affective Responses to Taste and Flavor: Top-Down Influences

on the Orbitofrontal and Pregenual Cingulate Cortices," *Cerebral Cortex* 18, no. 7 (July 2008): 1549–1559, http://doi.org/10.1093/cercor/bhm185.

15. B. P. Turnwald and A. J. Crum, "Smart Food Policy for Healthy Food Labeling: Leading with Taste, Not Healthiness, to Shift Consumption and Enjoyment of Healthy Foods," *Preventive Medicine* 119 (February 2019): 7–13, https://doi.org/10.1016/j.ypmed.2018.11.021.

CHAPTER 5. DECISION DISRUPTOR #2: REBELLION

1. Catherine Gray, *The Unexpected Joy of the Ordinary* (London: Aster, 2020), 218.

2. J. Dimmock et al., "Not All Promotion Is Good Promotion: The Pitfalls of Overexaggerted Claims and Controlling Language in Exercise Messaging," *Journal of Sport Exercise Psychology* 2 (January 2020), https://doi.org/10.1123/jsep.2019-0193.

3. B. D. Rosenberg and J. T. Siegel, "Threatening Uncertainty and Psychological Reactance: Are Freedom Threats Always Noxious?" *Current Psychology* (April 2021), https://doi.org/10.1007/s12144-021-01640-8.

4. E. Jonas et al., "Culture, Self and the Emergence of Reactance: Is There a 'Universal' Freedom?" *Journal of Experimental Social Psychology* 45 (2009): 1068–1080.

5. Y. Zemack-Rugar, S. G. Moore, and G. J. Fitzsimons, "Just Do It! Why Committed Consumers React Negatively to Assertive Ads," *Journal of Consumer Psychology* 27, no. 3 (July 2017): 287–301, https://doi.org/10.1016/j.jcps.2017.01.002.

C. Steindl et al., "Understanding Psychological Reactance: New Developments and Findings," *Zeitschrift fur Psychologie–Journal of Psychology* 223, no. 4 (2015): 205–214.

Jack W. Brehm, *A Theory of Psychological Reactance* (Cambridge: Academic Press, 1966).

6. R. Thaler, "Nudges—What's Next for Nudging and Choice Architecture?" *Organizational Behavior and Human Decision Processes* 163 (March 2021): 4–5.

7. Mindset 2021, conference by Omada Health (April 14–15, 2021), https://summit.omadahealth.com/.

8. J. La Guardia and A. Bucher, "Nudges Are Not Enough to Propel Your Population," session at the Omada Health Mindset 2021 conference (April 15, 2021).

9. Zemack-Rugar, Moore, and Fitzsimons, "Just Do It!"

M. Dewies et al., "Nudging Is Ineffective When Attitudes Are Unsupportive: An Example from a Natural Field Experiment," *Basic and Applied Social Psychology* (May 2021), https://doi.org/10.1080/01973533.2021.1917412.

10. La Guardia and Bucher, "Nudges Are Not Enough to Propel Your Population."

11. Steindl et al., "Understanding Psychological Reactance."

12. Steindl et al., "Understanding Psychological Reactance."

13. L. Festinger and J. M. Carlsmith, "Cognitive Consequences of Forced Compliance," *Journal of Abnormal and Social Psychology* 58, no. 2 (1959): 203–210.

14. K. M. Sheldon and L. Houser-Marko, "Self-Concordance, Goal-Attainment, and the Pursuit of Happiness: Can There Be an Upward Spiral?" *Journal of Personality and Social Psychology* 80 (2001): 152–165.

Edward L. Deci and Richard M. Ryan, eds., *Handbook of Self-Determination Research* (Rochester, NY: University of Rochester Press, 2002).

Richard M. Ryan and Edward L. Deci, *Self-Determination Theory: Basic Psychological Needs in Motivation, Development, and Wellness* (New York: Guilford Press, 2017).

15. Jennifer Taber, phone interview, May 30, 2021.

16. S. W. Flint, J. Raisborough, and J. Hudson, "Editorial: The Implications of Weight Bias Internalization," *Frontiers in Psychology* 14 (January 2020), https://doi.org/10.3389/fpsyg.2019.03019.

L. E. Hayward, L. R. Vartanian, and R. T. Pinkus, "Weight Stigma Predicts Poorer Psychological Well-Being Through Internalized Weight Bias and Maladaptive Coping Responses," *Obesity* 26 (2018): 755–761, https://doi.org/10.1002/oby.22126.

A. J. Tomiyama et al., "How and Why Weight Stigma Drives the Obesity 'Epidemic' and Harms Health," *BMC Medicine* 16, no. 123 (2018), https://doi.org/10.1186/s12916-018-1116-5.

A. J. Tomiyama, "Stress and Obesity," *Annual Review of Psychology* 70 (2019): 703–718.

17. O. Williams and E. Annandale, "Weight Bias Internalization as an Embodied Process: Understanding How Obesity Stigma Gets Under the Skin," *Frontiers in Psychology* 10, no. 953 (April 29, 2019): 1–5.

18. Williams and Annandale, "Weight Bias Internalization."

19. M. L. Segar, J. S. Eccles, and C. R. Richardson, "Type of Physical Activity Goal Influences Participation in Healthy Midlife Women," *Women's Health Issues* 18, no. 4 (2008): 281–291.

M. L. Segar et al., "Midlife Women's Physical Activity Goals: Sociocultural Influences and Effects on Behavioral Regulation," *Sex Roles* 57, no. 11/12 (2007): 837–850.

E. Mailey et al., "Goals Matter: Exercising for Well-Being but Not Health or Appearance Predicts Future Exercise Behavior Among Parents," *Journal of Physical Activity and Health* 15, no. 11 (2018): 857–865.

20. Tomiyama et al., "How and Why Weight Stigma Drives the Obesity 'Epidemic.'"

CHAPTER 6. DECISION DISRUPTOR #3: ACCOMMODATION

1. P. J. Teixeira et al., "Motivation, Self-Determination, and Long-Term Weight Control," *International Journal of Behavioral Nutrition and Physical Activity* 9, no. 22 (2012), https://doi.org/10.1186/1479-5868-9-22.

Richard M. Ryan and Edward L. Deci, *Self-Determination Theory: Basic Psychological Needs in Motivation, Development, and Wellness* (New York: Guilford Press, 2017).

R. M. Ryan et al., "Facilitating Health Behaviour Change and Its Maintenance: Interventions Based on Self-Determination Theory," *European Health Psychologist* 10 (2008): 2–5.

2. Dictionary.com, "Altruism," https://www.dictionary.com/browse/altruism.

3. R. Jorge, I. Santos, and V. H. Teixeira, "Does Diet Strictness Level During Weekends and Holiday Periods Influence 1-Year Follow-Up Weight Loss Maintenance? Evidence from the Portuguese Weight Control Registry," *Nutrition Journal* 18, no. 3 (January 11, 2019).

A. Joki, J. Makela, and M. Fogelholm, "Permissive Flexibility in Successful Lifelong Weight Management: A Qualitative Study Among Finnish Men and Women," *Appetite* 116 (September 2017): 157–163.

4. Adam M. Grant, *Give and Take: Why Helping Others Drives Our Success* (London: Penguin Books, 2014).

5. S. L. Brown and R. M. Brown, "Connecting Prosocial Behavior to Improved Physical Health: Contributions from the Neurobiology of Parenting," *Neuroscience & Biobehavioral Reviews* 55 (August 2015): 1–17.

R. N. Lawton et al., "Does Volunteering Make Us Happier, or Are Happier People More Likely to Volunteer? Addressing the Problem of Reverse Causality When Estimating the Wellbeing Impacts of Volunteering," *Journal of Happiness Studies* 22 (2021): 599–624.

Cleveland Clinic.org, "Why Giving Is Good for Your Health" (October 28, 2020), https://health.clevelandclinic.org/why-giving-is-good-for-your-health/.

6. A. Grant and R. Rebele, "Beat Generosity Burnout," *Harvard Business Review*, (January 23, 2017), https://hbr.org/2017/01/beat-generosity-burnout.

7. V. S. Helgeson and H. L. Fritz, "A Theory of Unmitigated Communion," *Personality and Social Psychology Review* 2, no. 3 (1998): 173–183.

8. S. B. Kaufman and E. Jauk, "Healthy Selfishness and Pathological Altruism: Measuring Two Paradoxical Forms of Selfishness," *Frontiers in Psychology* 11, no. 1006 (2020), https://doi.org10.3389/fpsyg.2020.01006.

9. V. S. Helgeson et al., "Psychosocial Predictors of Diabetes Risk Factors and Complications: An 11-Year Follow-Up," *Health Psychology* 38, no. 7, (July 2019): 567–576, https://doi.org/10.1037/hea0000730.

10. Adam Grant, "Successful Givers, Toxic Takers, and the Life We Spend at Work," *On Being with Krista Tippett* (podcast), https://onbeing.org/programs/adam-grant-successful-givers-toxic-takers-and-the-life-we-spend-at-work/.

11. C. M. Barnes et al., "Leader Sleep Devaluation, Employee Sleep, and Unethical Behavior," *Sleep Health* 6, no. 3 (June 2020), http://doi.org10.1016/j.sleh.2019.12.001.

12. Gretchen Spreitzer, personal communication (email), June 6, 2021.

13. C. Barnes, "Sleep-Deprived People Are More Likely to Cheat," *Harvard Business Review* (May 31, 2013), https://hbr.org/2013/05/sleep-deprived-people-are-more-likely-to-cheat.

14. C. M. Barnes et al., "'You Wouldn't Like Me When I'm Sleepy': Leaders' Sleep, Daily Abusive Supervision, and Work Unit Engagement,"

Academy of Management Journal 58, no. 5 (November 3, 2014), https://doi .org/10.5465/amj.2013.1063.

15. M. Segar et al., "Rethinking Physical Activity Communication: Using Qualitative Methods to Understand Women's Goals, Values, and Beliefs to Improve Public Health," *BMC Public Health* 17, no. 462 (2017), https://doi .org/10.1186/s12889-017-4361-1.

16. Tara Parker Pope, "Why Self-Care Isn't Selfish," *New York Times*, January 6, 2021, https://www.nytimes.com/2021/01/06/well/live/why -self-care-isnt-selfish.html.

CHAPTER 7. DECISION DISRUPTOR #4: PERFECTION

1. S. R. Locke and L. R. Brawley, "Development and Initial Validity of the Exercise-Related Cognitive Errors Questionnaire," *Psychology of Sport and Exercise* 23 (2016): 82–89, https://doi.org/10.1016/j.psychsport.2015 .11.003.

2. S. R. Locke and L. R. Brawley, "Perceptions of Exercise Consistency: Relation to Exercise-Related Cognitive Errors and Cognitions," *Journal of Health Psychology* 22, no. 5 (April 2017): 684–694, https://doi .org/10.1177/1359105315611956.

3. K. L. Piercy et al., "The Physical Activity Guidelines for Americans," *JAMA* 320, no. 19 (November 2018): 2020–2028, http://doi.org/10.1001 /jama.2018.14854, PMID: 30418471.

4. F. C. Bull et al., "World Health Organization 2020 Guidelines on Physical Activity and Sedentary Behaviour," *British Journal of Sports Medicine* 54, no. 24 (December 2020): 1451–1462, https://doi.org/10.1136 /bjsports-2020-102955.

5. Health.gov, "Move Your Way Campaign," accessed September 13, 2020, https://health.gov/our-work/physical-activity/move-your-way-campaign.

6. SportEngland.org, "This Girl Can," accessed October 13, 2020, https:// www.sportengland.org/campaigns-and-our-work/this-girl-can.

7. Sigaoassobio.pt, "A atividade física chama por si," accessed October 13, 2020, https://www.sigaoassobio.pt/pt.

8. M. L. Segar et al., "Everything Counts in Sending the Right Message: Science-Based Messaging Implications from the 2020 WHO Guidelines on

Physical Activity and Sedentary Behaviour," *International Journal of Behavioral Nutrition and Physical Activity* 17, no. 1 (November 4, 2020): 135, https://doi.org/10.1186/s12966-020-01048-w.

9. C. Duarte et al., "What Makes Dietary Restraint Problematic? Development and Validation of the Inflexible Eating Questionnaire," *Appetite* 114 (2017): 146–154, ISSN 0195-6663, https://doi.org/10.1016/j.appet.2017.03.034.

10. Brent Darden, personal communication, June 9, 2021.

11. H. B. Kappes and G. Oettingen, "Positive Fantasies About Idealized Futures Sap Energy," *Journal of Experimental Social Psychology* 47, no. 4 (2011): 719–729, ISSN 0022-1031.

12. L. Uziel and R. F. Baumeister, "The Self-Control Irony: Desire for Self-Control Limits Exertion of Self-Control in Demanding Settings," *Personality and Social Psychology Bulletin* 43, no. 5 (May 2017): 693–705, http://doi.org/10.1177/0146167217695555.

CHAPTER 8. THE JOY CHOICE: THE PERFECT *IMPERFECT* OPTION

1. F. F. Sniehotta, U. Scholz, and R. Schwarzer, "Action Plans and Coping Plans for Physical Exercise: A Longitudinal Intervention Study in Cardiac Rehabilitation," *British Journal of Health Psychology* 11, pt. 1 (February 2006): 23–37, http://doi.org/10.1348/135910705X43804.

R. B. Lopez et al., "Associations Between Use of Self-Regulatory Strategies and Daily Eating Patterns: An Experience Sampling Study in College-Aged Women," *Motivation and Emotion* (July 2021), https://doi.org/10.1007/s11031-021-09903-4.

S. P. Goldstein et al., "Identifying Behavioral Types of Dietary Lapse from a Mobile Weight Loss Program: Preliminary Investigation from a Secondary Data Analysis," *Appetite* (November 2021): 166, https://doi.org/10.1016/j.appet.2021.105440.

2. F. Shaddy, A. Fishbach, and I. Simonson, "Trade-Offs in Choice," *Annual Review of Psychology* 4, no. 72 (January 2021): 181–206, https://doi.org/10.1146/annurev-psych-072420-125709.

3. M. Segar et al., "Rethinking Physical Activity Communication: Using Focus Groups to Understand Women's Goals, Values, and Beliefs to Improve

Public Health," *BMC Public Health* 17, no. 1 (May 2017): 462, http://doi
.org/10.1186/s12889-017-4361-1.

4. J. T. Nigg, "Annual Research Review: On the Relations Among Self-
Regulation, Self-Control, Executive Functioning, Effortful Control, Cognitive Control, Impulsivity, Risk-Taking, and Inhibition for Developmental
Psychopathology," *Journal of Child Psychology and Psychiatry, and Allied Disciplines* 58, no. 4 (2017): 361–383, https://doi.org/10.1111/jcpp.12675.

5. A. Diamond, "Executive Functions," *Annual Review of Psychology* 64
(2013): 135–168, https://doi.org/10.1146/annurev-psych-113011-1437.

C. C. Raver and C. Blair, "Neuroscientific Insights: Attention, Working
Memory, and Inhibitory Control." *Future of Children* 26, no. 2 (2016): 95–
118, http://www.jstor.org/stable/43940583.

Nigg, "Annual Research Review."

6. E. T. Berkman, "The Neuroscience of Goals and Behavior Change,"
Journal of Consulting and Clinical Psychology 70, no. 1 (March 2018): 28–44,
http://doi.org/10.1037/cpb0000094.

7. Berkman, "The Neuroscience of Goals and Behavior Change."

CHAPTER 9. SIMPLIFY: SUPPORTING WORKING MEMORY

1. W. Hofmann et al., "Working Memory Capacity and Self-Regulatory
Behavior: Toward an Individual Differences Perspective on Behavior Determination by Automatic Versus Controlled Processes," *Journal of Personality and Social Psychology* 95, no. 4 (October 2008): 962–977, http://doi
.org/10.1037/a0012705.

2. Alex Burmester, "Working Memory: How You Keep Things 'in Mind'
over the Short Term," *The Conversation* (June 4, 2017), https://theconversa
tion.com/profiles/alex-burmester-197396.

3. E. J. Adams, A. T. Nguyen, and N. Cowan, "Theories of Working
Memory: Differences in Definition, Degree of Modularity, Role of Attention, and Purpose," *Language, Speech, and Hearing Services in Schools* 49, no. 3
(2018): 340–355, https://doi.org/10.1044/2018_LSHSS-17-0114.

4. Joel Nigg, personal communication (email), April 14, 2021.

5. L. F. Barrett, M. M. Tugade, and R. W. Engle, "Individual Differences in
Working Memory Capacity and Dual-Process Theories of the Mind," *Psycho-

logical Bulletin 130, no. 4 (2004): 553–573, https://doi.org/10.1037/0033 -2909.130.4.553.

6. C. R. Brewin and L. Smart, "Working Memory Capacity and Suppression of Intrusive Thoughts," *Journal of Behavior Therapy and Experimental Psychiatry* 36, no. 1 (March 2005): 61–68, http://doi.org/10.1016/j.jbtep.2004.11.006.

7. K. Tapper, "Mindfulness and Craving: Effects and Mechanisms," *Clinical Psychology Review* 59 (February 2018): 101–117, http://doi.org/10.1016/j .cpr.2017.11.003.

8. W. Hofmann, B. J. Schmeichel, and A. D. Baddeley, "Executive Functions and Self-Regulation Trends," *Cognitive Science* 16, no. 3 (March 2012): 174–180, http://doi.org10.1016/j.tics.2012.01.006.

S. Dohle, K. Diel, and W. Hofmann, "Executive Functions and the Self-Regulation of Eating Behavior: A Review," *Appetite* 1, no. 124 (May 2018): 4–9, http://doi.org10.1016/j.appet.2017.05.041.

9. John Ratey, personal communication (email). June 26, 2021.

10. John J. Ratey, *SPARK: The Revolutionary New Science of Exercise and the Brain* (New York: Little Brown, 2013).

Y. Yamazaki et al., "Inter-individual Differences in Working Memory Improvement After Acute Mild and Moderate Aerobic Exercise," *PLoS One* 13, no. 12 (December 31, 2018): e0210053, http:// doi.org/10.1371/journal .pone.0210053.

11. Edward M. Hallowell and John J. Ratey, *ADHD 2.0: New Science and Essential Strategies for Thriving with Distraction—from Childhood Through Adulthood* (New York: Ballantine Books, 2021).

Joel Nigg, *Getting Ahead of ADHD: What Next-Generation Science Says About Treatments That Work—and How You Can Make Them Work for Your Child* (New York: Guilford Press, 2017).

12. Ratey, *SPARK*.

13. Hofmann et al., "Working Memory Capacity and Self-Regulatory Behavior."

14. Ratey, *SPARK*.

15. Lumosity, "Brain Training Built on Science," https://www.lumosity .com/en/science/.

16. J. L. Hardy et al., "Enhancing Cognitive Abilities with Comprehensive Training: A Large, Online, Randomized, Active-Controlled Trial,"

PLoS One 5, no. 7 (September 2, 2015), https://doi.org/10.1371/journal .pone.0134467.

17. N. J. Gates et al., "Computerised Cognitive Training for 12 or More Weeks for Maintaining Cognitive Function in Cognitively Healthy People in Late Life," *Cochrane Database of Systematic Reviews* 2, no. CD012277 (2020), https://doi.org/10.1002/14651858.

Anjana Ahuja, "An Evidence Deficit Haunts the Billion-Dollar Brain Training Industry," *Financial Times*, January 23, 2019, https://www.ft.com /content/a0166eea-1e41-11e9-a46f-08f9738d6b2b.

18. J. F. Vermeir et al., "The Effects of Gamification on Computerized Cognitive Training: Systematic Review and Meta-analysis," *JMIR Serious Games* 8, no. 3 (August 10, 2020): e18644, http://doi.org/10.2196 /18644.

19. F. C. M. Dassen et al., "Gamified Working Memory Training in Overweight Individuals Reduces Food Intake but Not Body Weight," *Appetite* 1, no. 124 (May 2018): 89–98, http://doi.org/10.1016/j.appet.2017.05 .009.

V. Whitelock et al., "Does Working Memory Training Improve Dietary Self-Care in Type 2 Diabetes Mellitus? Results of a Double Blind Randomised Controlled Trial," *Diabetes Research and Clinical Practice* 143 (September 2018): 204–214, http://doi.org/10.1016/j.diabres.2018.07.005.

20. Julie Dirksen, *Design for How People Learn*, 2nd ed. (San Francisco: New Riders, 2015).

21. N. Cowan, "Working Memory Underpins Cognitive Development, Learning, and Education," *Educational Psychology Review* 26, no. 2 (2014): 197–223, https://doi.org/10.1007/s10648-013-9246-y.

22. Dirksen, *Design for How People Learn*.

23. Julie Dirksen, personal communication (email), August 24, 2021.

24. Joshua Foer, *Moonwalking with Einstein: The Art and Science of Remembering Everything* (London: Penguin Press, 2011).

25. N. A. Kompa and J. L. Mueller, "How Abstract (Non-embodied) Linguistic Representations Augment Cognitive Control," *Frontiers in Psychology* 11 (2020): 1597, https://doi.org/10.3389/fpsyg.2020.01597.

CHAPTER 10. PLAY: SUPPORTING FLEXIBLE THINKING

1. K. A. Carr and L. H. Epstein, "Choice Is Relative: Reinforcing Value of Food and Activity in Obesity Treatment," *American Psychologist Journal* 75, no. 2 (February–March 2020): 139–151, http://doi.org/10.1037/amp0000521.

2. B. D. Sylvester et al., "Is Variety a Spice of (an Active) Life?: Perceived Variety, Exercise Behavior, and the Mediating Role of Autonomous Motivation," *Journal of Sport and Exercise Psychology* 36, no. 5 (October 2014): 516–527, http://doi.org/10.1123/jsep.2014-0102.

3. Wikipedia, "Play," https://en.wikipedia.org/wiki/Play_(activity).

4. D. Bondi and D. Bondi, "Free Play or Not Free Play: An Interdisciplinary Approach to Deal with Paradoxes," *Creativity Research Journal* 33, no. 1 (2020): 26–32, https://doi.org/10.1080/10400419.2020.1833543.

5. J. Beddington et al., "The Mental Wealth of Nations," *Nature* 455 (2008): 1057–1060, https://doi.org/10.1038/4551057a.

Leonard Mlodinow, *Elastic: Unlocking Your Brain's Ability to Embrace Change* (New York: Vintage Books, 2018).

6. T. B. Kashdan and J. Rottenberg, "Psychological Flexibility as a Fundamental Aspect of Health," *Clinical Psychology Review* 30, no. 7 (November 2010): 865–878, http://doi.org/10.1016/j.cpr.2010.03.001A.

G. Usubini et al., "The Impact of Psychological Flexibility on Psychological Well-Being in Adults with Obesity," *Frontiers in Psychology* 12 (March 22, 2021): 636933, http://doi.org/10.3389/fpsyg.2021.636933.

7. J. T. Nigg, "Annual Research Review: On the Relations Among Self-Regulation, Self-Control, Executive Functioning, Effortful Control, Cognitive Control, Impulsivity, Risk-Taking, and Inhibition for Developmental Psychopathology," *Journal of Child Psychology and Psychiatry* 58, no. 4 (April 2017): 361–383, http://doi.org/10.1111/jcpp.12675.

8. E. Sairanen et al., "Flexibility in Weight Management," *Eating Behaviors* 15, no. 2 (April 2014): 218–224, http://doi.org/10.1016/j.eatbeh.2014.01.008.

P. J. Teixeira et al., "Successful Behavior Change in Obesity Interventions in Adults: A Systematic Review of Self-Regulation Mediators," *BMC*

Medicine 16, no. 13 (April 2015): 84, http://doi.org/10.1186/s12916-015 -0323-6.

M. L. Segar et al., "From a Vital Sign to Vitality: Selling Exercise So Patients Want to Buy It," *Translational Journal of the American College of Sports Medicine* 1, no. 11 (2016): 97–102.

M. L. Segar et al., "Everything Counts in Sending the Right Message: Science-Based Messaging Implications from the 2020 WHO Guidelines on Physical Activity and Sedentary Behaviour," *International Journal of Behavioral Nutrition and Physical Activity* 17, no. 135 (2020), https://doi .org/10.1186/s12966-020-01048-w.

9. Society for Adolescent Health and Medicine, "Preventing Nutritional Disorders in Adolescents by Encouraging a Healthy Relationship with Food," *Journal of Adolescent Health* 67, no. 6 (December 2020): 875–879, http://doi.org/10.1016/j.jadohealth.2020.09.022. PMID: 33220798.

10. R. Y. Arends et al., "The Longitudinal Relation Between Patterns of Goal Management and Psychological Health in People with Arthritis: The Need for Adaptive Flexibility," *British Journal of Health Psychology* 21, no. 2 (May 2016): 469–489, https://doi.org10.1111/bjhp.12182.

11. D. Kwasnicka, N. Ntoumanis, and F. F. Sniehotta, "Setting Performance and Learning Goals Is Useful for Active and Inactive Individuals, If Goals Are Personalized and Flexible: Commentary on Swann et al. (2020)," *Health Psychology Review* 15, no. 1 (March 2021): 51–55, http://doi.org/10 .1080/17437199.2020.1762107.

12. S. Dohle, K. Diel, and W. Hofmann, "Executive Functions and the Self-regulation of Eating Behavior: A Review," *Appetite* 1, no. 124 (May 2018): 4–9, http://doi.org/10.1016/j.appet.2017.05.041.

A. Joki, J. Mäkelä, and M. Fogelholm, "Permissive Flexibility in Successful Lifelong Weight Management: A Qualitative Study Among Finnish Men and Women," *Appetite* 1, no. 116 (September 2017): 157–163, http:// doi.org/10.1016/j.appet.2017.04.031.

13. Teixeira et al., "Successful Behavior Change."

14. R. Jorge et al., "Does Diet Strictness Level During Weekends and Holiday Periods Influence 1-Year Follow-Up Weight Loss Maintenance? Evidence from the Portuguese Weight Control Registry," *Nutrition Journal* 18, no. 1 (2019): 3, https://doi.org/10.1186/s12937-019-0430-x.

15. S. M. Kelly and J. A. Updegraff, "Substituting Activities Mediates the Effect of Cognitive Flexibility on Physical Activity: A Daily Diary Study," *Journal of Behavioral Medicine* 40, no. 4 (August 2017): 669–674, http:// doi.org/10.1007/s10865-017-9839-x.

16. J. Andrade et al., "Use of a Clay Modeling Task to Reduce Chocolate Craving," *Appetite* 58, no. 3 (June 2012): 955–963, http://doi.org/10.1016/j .appet.2012.02.044K.

K. Tapper, "Mindfulness and Craving: Effects and Mechanisms," *Clinical Psychology Review* 59 (2018): 101–117, http://doi.org/10.1016/j.cpr .2017.11.003.

17. T. B. Kashdan and M. F. Steger, "Curiosity and Pathways to Well-Being and Meaning in Life: Traits, States, and Everyday Behaviors," *Motivation and Emotion* 31, no. 3 (2007): 159–173, https://doi.org/10.1007 /s11031-007-9068-7.

D. Grigorescu, "Curiosity, Intrinsic Motivation and the Pleasure of Knowledge," *Journal of Educational Sciences & Psychology* 10, no. 1 (2020): 16–23.

B. L. Fredrickson, "The Broaden-and-Build Theory of Positive Emotions," *Philosophical Transactions of the Royal Society B: Biological Sciences* 359, no. 1449 (September 29, 2004): 1367–1378, http://doi.10.1098 /rstb.2004.1512.

18. N. S. Schutte and J. M. Malouff, "Increasing Curiosity Through Autonomy of Choice," *Motivation and Emotion* 43 (2019): 563–570, https:// doi.org/10.1007/s11031-019-09758-w.

19. B. L. Fredrickson and T. Joiner, "Reflections on Positive Emotions and Upward Spirals," *Perspectives on Psychological Science* 13, no. 2 (March 2018): 194–199, http://doi.org/10.1177/1745691617692106, PMID: 29592643, PMCID: PMC5877808.

20. S. Liu, "Broaden the Mind Before Ideation: The Effect of Conceptual Attention Scope on Creativity," *Thinking Skills and Creativity* 22 (2016): 190–200, https://doi.org/10.1016/j.tsc.2016.10.004.

21. R. F. Baumeister, H. M. Maranges, and H. Sjåstad, "Consciousness of the Future as a Matrix of Maybe: Pragmatic Prospection and the Simulation of Alternative Possibilities," *Psychology of Consciousness: Theory, Research, and Practice* 5, no. 3 (2018): 223–238, https://doi.org/10.1037/cns0000154.

22. Carr and Epstein, "Choice Is Relative."

CHAPTER 11. CHOOSE JOY: SUPPORTING INHIBITION

1. J. T. Nigg, "Annual Research Review: On the Relations Among Self-Regulation, Self-Control, Executive Functioning, Effortful Control, Cognitive Control, Impulsivity, Risk-Taking, and Inhibition for Developmental Psychopathology," *Journal of Child Psychology and Psychiatry* 58, no. 4 (April 2017): 361–383, http://doi.org/10.1111/jcpp.12675.

2. L. Uziel and R. F. Baumeister, "The Self-Control Irony: Desire for Self-Control Limits Exertion of Self-Control in Demanding Settings," *Personality and Social Psychology Bulletin* 43, no. 5 (May 2017): 693–705, https://doi.org/10.1177/0146167217695555.

3. J. Y. Shah, R. Friedman, and A. W. Kruglanski, "Forgetting All Else: On the Antecedents and Consequences of Goal Shielding," *Journal of Personality and Social Psychology* 83, no. 6 (December 2002): 1261–1280.

4. PsyToolkit, "Go.No-Go Task," https://www.psytoolkit.org/experiment-library/go-no-go.html.

5. V. Allom, B. Mullan, and M. Hagger, "Does Inhibitory Control Training Improve Health Behaviour? A Meta-analysis," *Health Psychology Review* 10, no. 2 (June 2016): 168–186, http://doi.org/ 10.1080/17437199.2015.1051078.

6. E. M. Forman et al., "Promising Technological Innovations in Cognitive Training to Treat Eating-Related Behavior," *Appetite* 1, no. 124 (May 2018): 68–77, https://doi.org/10.1016/j.appet.2017.04.01.

A. L. Miller et al., "Targeting Self-Regulation to Promote Health Behaviors in Children," *Behaviour Research and Therapy* 101 (February 2018): 71–81, https://doi.org/10.1016/j.brat.2017.09.008.

7. M. Segar et al., "Rethinking Physical Activity Communication: Using Focus Groups to Understand Women's Goals, Values, and Beliefs to Improve Public Health," *BMC Public Health* 17, no. 1 (May 2017): 462, https://doi.org/10.1186/s12889-017-4361-1.

8. M. L. Segar, J. S. Eccles, and C. Richardson, "Rebranding Exercise: Closing the Gap Between Values and Behavior," *International Journal of Behavioral Nutrition and Physical Activity* 8 (2011): 94.

M. L. Segar et al., "Fitting Fitness into Women's Lives: Effects of a Gender-Tailored Physical Activity Intervention," *Women's Health Issues* 12 (2002): 338–347.

C. J. Stevens and A. D. Bryan, "A Case for Leveraging Integrated Regulation Strategies to Optimize Health Benefits from Self-Determined Exercise Behavior," *Annals of Behavioral Medicine* 49, no. 5 (October 2015): 783–784, https://doi.org/10.1007/s12160-015-9722-3.

M. Quirin et al., "Effortless Willpower? The Integrative Self and Self-Determined Goal Pursuit," *Frontiers in Psychology* 12 (March 18, 2021): 653458, http://doi.org/10.3389/fpsyg.2021.653458.

9. E. T. Berkman, "Value-Based Choice: An Integrative, Neuroscience-Informed Model of Health Goals," *Psychology & Health* 33, no. 1 (January 2018): 40–57, https://doi.org/10.1080/08870446.2017.1316847.

10. Berkman, "Value-Based Choice."

Quirin et al., "Effortless Willpower?"

11. E. B. Falk et al., "Neural Bases of Affirmation," *Proceedings of the National Academy of Sciences*, 201500247 (February 2015), https://doi.org/10.1073/pnas.1500247112.

12. Emily Falk, personal communication (email), August 9, 2021.

13. J. K. Dominick and S. Cole, "Goals as Identities: Boosting Perceptions of Healthy-Eater Identity for Easier Goal Pursuit," *Motivation and Emotion* 44 (2020): 410–426, https://doi.org/10.1007/s11031-020-09824-8.

14. Quirin et al., "Effortless Willpower?"

15. Berkman, "Value-Based Choice."

A. Wigfield and J. S. Eccles, "Expectancy-Value Theory of Achievement Motivation," *Contemporary Educational Psychology* 25, no. 1 (January 2000): 68–81, http://doi.org/10.1006/ceps.1999.1015.

16. G. Brand and P. Ekkekakis, "Affective–Reflective Theory of Physical Inactivity and Exercise," *German Journal of Exercise and Sport Research* 48 (2018): 48–58, https://doi.org/10.1007/s12662-017-0477-9.

J. A. Brewer et al., "Can Mindfulness Address Maladaptive Eating Behaviors? Why Traditional Diet Plans Fail and How New Mechanistic Insights May Lead to Novel Interventions," *Frontiers in Psychology* 9 (September 2018): 1418, http://doi.org/10.3389/fpsyg.2018.01418.

17. Brewer et al., "Can Mindfulness Address Maladaptive Eating Behaviors?"

18. W. Hofman et al., "The Spoiled Pleasure of Giving In to Temptation," *Motivation and Emotion* 13 (2013): 733–742, https://doi.org/10.1007/s11031-013-9355-4.

19. M. L. Segar et al., "Fitting Fitness into Women's Lives: Effects of a Gender-Tailored Physical Activity Intervention," *Women's Health Issues* 12 (2002): 338–347.

Michelle Segar, *No Sweat: How the Simple Science of Motivation Can Bring You a Lifetime of Fitness* (New York: Amacom, 2015).

P. J. Teixeira et al., "Exercise, Physical Activity, and Self-Determination Theory: A Systematic Review," *International Journal of Behavioral Nutrition and Physical Activity* 9, no. 78 (2012), https://doi.org/10.1186/1479 -5868-9-78.

20. R. E. Rhodes and A. Kates, "Can the Affective Response to Exercise Predict Future Motives and Physical Activity Behavior? A Systematic Review of Published Evidence," *Annals of Behavioral Medicine* 49 (2015): 715–731.

21. M. N. Shiota et al., "Positive Affect and Behavior Change," *Current Opinion in Behavioral Sciences* 39 (2021): 222–228.

E. K. Papies et al., "Using Consumption and Reward Simulations to Increase the Appeal of Plant-Based Foods," *Appetite* 155 (2020), https:// doi.org/10.1016/j.appet.2020.104812.

K. Woolley and A. Fishbach, "For the Fun of It: Harnessing Immediate Rewards to Increase Persistence in Long-Term Goals," *Journal of Consumer Research* 42, no. 6 (April 2016): 952–966, https://doi.org/10.1093/jcr /ucv098.

22. S. Doebel, "Rethinking Executive Function and Its Development," *Perspectives on Psychological Science* 15, no. 4 (July 2020): 942–956, https:// doi.org/10.1177/1745691620904771.

A. E. Caldwell et al., "Harnessing Centred Identity Transformation to Reduce Executive Function Burden for Maintenance of Health Behaviour Change: The Maintain IT Model," *Healthy Psychology Review* 12, no. 3 (September 2018): 231–253, https://doi.org/10.1080/17437199.2018.14 37551.

23. J. D. Creswell et al., "Self-Affirmation Improves Problem-Solving Under Stress," *PLoS One* 8, no. 5 (May 2013): e62593, https://doi.org /10.1371/journal.pone.0062593.

P. S. Harris, P. R. Harris, and E. Miles, "Self-Affirmation Improves Performance on Tasks Related to Executive Functioning," *Journal of Experi-*

mental Social Psychology 70 (2017): 281–285, https://doi.org/10.1016/j
.jesp.2016.11.011.

24. M. Segar et al., "Rethinking Physical Activity Communication."

B. L. Fredrickson and T. Joiner, "Reflections on Positive Emotions and
Upward Spirals," *Perspectives on Psychological Science* 13, no. 2 (March 2018):
194–199, http://doi.org/10.1177/1745691617692106, PMID: 29592643,
PMCID: PMC5877808.

M. L. Segar et al., "From a Vital Sign to Vitality: Selling Exercise So
Patients Want to Buy It," *Translational Journal of the American College of
Sports Medicine* 1, no. 11 (2016): 97–102.

25. Segar et al., "Fitting Fitness into Women's Lives."

J. M. Rogers, "Mindfulness-Based Interventions for Adults Who Are
Overweight or Obese: A Meta-analysis of Physical and Psychological
Health Outcomes," *Obesity Reviews* 18, no. 1 (January 2017): 51–67, http://
doi.org/10.1111/obr.12461.

Scott Barry Kaufman, *Transcend: The New Science of Self-Actualization*
(New York: TarcherPerigee, 2021).

M. L. Butryn, "Pilot Test of an Acceptance-Based Behavioral Intervention
to Promote Physical Activity During Weight Loss Maintenance," *Behavioral
Medicine* 44, no. 1 (January–March 2018): 77–87, http://doi.org/10.1080
/08964289.2016.1170663.

Victor J. Strecher, *Life on Purpose: How Living for What Matters Most
Changes Everything* (San Francisco: HarperOne, 2016).

CHAPTER 12. POP! THE JOY CHOICE DECISION TOOL AND HOW TO USE IT

1. Joshua Foer, *Moonwalking with Einstein: The Art and Science of Remembering Everything* (London: Penguin Press, 2011).

2. S. Hoffmann et al., "Keeping the Pace: The Effect of Slow-Paced
Breathing on Error Monitoring," *International Journal of Psychophysiology* 146
(December 2019): 217–224, http://doi.org10.1016/j.ijpsycho.2019.10.001.

3. V. U. Ludwig, K. W. Brown, and J. A. Brewer, "Self-Regulation Without Force: Can Awareness Leverage Reward to Drive Behavior Change?"
Perspectives in Psychological Science 15, no. 6 (November 2020): 1382–1399,
http://doi.org/10.1177/1745691620931460.

4. Ludwig, Brown, and Brewer, "Self-Regulation Without Force."

Daniel J. Siegel, *Aware: The Science and Practice of Presence—The Ground-breaking Meditation Practice* (New York: TarcherPerigee, 2018).

5. Joel Nigg, phone communication, August 25, 2021.

6. Ethan Kross, *Chatter: The Voice in Our Head and How to Harness It* (London: Penguin Random House UK, 2021).

C. R. Furman, E. Kross, and A. N. Gearhardt, "Distanced Self-Talk Enhances Goal Pursuit to Eat Healthier," *Clinical Psychological Science* 8, no. 2 (2020): 366–373, https://doi.org/10.1177/2167702619896366.

CHAPTER 13. LEARNING LASTING CHANGE

1. L. Wirz, M. Bogdanov, and L. Schwabe, "Habits Under Stress: Mechanistic Insights Across Different Types of Learning," *Current Opinion in Behavioral Sciences* 20 (2018): 9–16, https://doi.org/10.1016/j.cobeha.2017.08.009.

A. O. Ceceli and E. Tricomi, "Habits and Goals: A Motivational Perspective on Action Control," *Current Opinion in Behavioral Sciences* 20 (2018): 110–116, https://doi.org/10.1016/j.cobeha.2017.12.005.

2. E. T. Berkman, "The Neuroscience of Goals and Behavior Change," *Journal of Consulting and Clinical Psychology* 70, no. 1 (March 2018): 28–44, http://doi.org/10.1037/cpb0000094.

3. J. H. Flavell, "Metacognitive Aspects of Problem Solving," in *The Nature of Intelligence*, ed. L. B. Resnick (Hillsdale, NJ: Erlbaum, 1976): 231–236.

4. Flavell, "Metacognitive Aspects of Problem Solving."

Saundra Yancy McGuire, *Teach Students How to Learn* (Sterling, VA: Stylus Publishing, 2015), 16.

5. Susan A. Ambrose et al., *How Learning Works: Seven Research-Based Principles for Smart Teaching* (San Francisco: Jossey-Bass, 2010).

McGuire, *Teach Students How to Learn*.

6. N. Yannier et al., "Active Learning: 'Hands-On' Meets 'Minds-On'," *Science* 374, no. 6563 (October 2021): 26–30.

7. Julie Dirksen, *Design for How People Learn*, 2nd ed. (San Francisco: New Riders, 2015).

APPENDIX A: GETTING STARTED PICKING THE JOY CHOICE: AN EATING EXAMPLE

1. K. Y. Wang, M. G. Bublitz, and G. T. Zhao, "Enhancing Dieters' Perseverance in Adversity: How Counterfactual Thinking Increases Use of Digital Health Tracking Tools," *Appetite* 164 (2021): 105261, https://doi.org/10.1016/j.appet.2021.105261.

2. C. Thøgersen-Ntoumani et al., "Does Self-Compassion Help to Deal with Dietary Lapses Among Overweight and Obese Adults Who Pursue Weight-Loss Goals?" *British Journal of Health Psychology* 26, no. 3 (September 2021): 767–788, http://doi.org/10.1111/bjhp.12499.

3. Tom Rath, *The Rechargeables: Eat Move Sleep* (Arlington, VA: Missionday, 2015), https://tomrath.org.

4. Maryann Jacobsen, *How to Raise a Mindful Eater: 8 Powerful Principles for Transforming Your Child's Relationship with Food* (CreateSpace Independent Publishing Platform, 2016), https://maryannjacobsen.com/books/.

5. Michelle Segar.com.

6. Evelyn Tribole and Elyse Resch, *Intuitive Eating: A Revolutionary Anti-Diet Approach*, 4th ed. (Ashland, OR: Blackstone Publishing, 2021).

7. Michelle Segar, *No Sweat: How the Simple Science of Motivation Can Bring You a Lifetime of Fitness* (New York: Anacom, 2015).

8. Daniel J. Siegel and Tina Payne Bryson, *The Yes Brain: How to Cultivate Courage, Curiosity, and Resilience in Your Child* (New York: Bantam, 2019).

9. William Ury, *Getting to Yes with Yourself: How to Get What You Truly Want* (San Francisco: HarperOne, 2016).

APPENDIX B: PROFESSIONAL GOALS AND INDUSTRY CASES

1. Brent Darden, personal communication (email), September 1, 2021.

2. Sara Hodson, personal communication (email), September 24, 2021.

3. D. Fave et al., "Sources and Motives for Personal Meaning in Adulthood," *Journal of Positive Psychology* 8, no. 6 (2013): 517–529.

C. Stevinson, G. Wiltshire, and M. Hickson, "Facilitating Participation in Health-Enhancing Physical Activity: A Qualitative Study of Parkrun," *International Journal of Behavioral Medicine* 22, no. 2 (2015): 170–177.

A. W. Kinsey et al., "Positive Outliers Among African American Women and the Factors Associated with Long-Term Physical Activity Maintenance," *Racial and Ethnic Health Disparities* 6 (2019): 603–617, https://doi.org/10.1007/s40615-018-00559-4.

4. Amy Bantham, personal communication (email), October 17, 2021.

5. LuAnn Heinen, personal communication (email), August 9, 2021.

6. Laura Putnam, personal communication (email), September 28, 2021.

7. Putnam.

8. Institute of Medicine, *Crossing the Quality Chasm: A New Health System for the 21st Century* (Washington, DC: National Academies Press, 2001).

9. S. J. Kuipers, J. M. Cramm, and A. P. Nieboer, "The Importance of Patient-Centered Care and Co-creation of Care for Satisfaction with Care and Physical and Social Well-Being of Patients with Multi-morbidity in the Primary Care Setting," *BMC Health Services Research* 19, no. 13 (2019), https://doi.org/10.1186/s12913-018-3818-y.

10. V. M. Montori, J. P. Brito, and M. H. Murad, "The Optimal Practice of Evidence-Based Medicine: Incorporating Patient Preferences in Practice Guidelines," *JAMA* 310 (2013): 2503–2504.

11. Victor Montori, personal communication (email), August 31, 2021.

12. M. L. Segar et al., "From a Vital Sign to Vitality: Selling Exercise So Patients Want to Buy It," *Translational Journal of the American College of Sports Medicine* 1, no. 11 (2016): 97–102.

13. Cindy Lin, personal communication (email), September 13, 2021.

DISCUSSION GUIDE QUESTIONS

I designed these questions to highlight some major themes of *THE JOY CHOICE* in order to help readers understand them more deeply personally and assist with making more sustainable healthy eating and exercise choices in their own life. I love hearing how my work is impacting people's lives. In addition to this Discussion Guide, you can learn more about *The Joy Choice*, access further information, or share your experiences with me by visiting michellesegar.com.

1. Do you agree with the idea that it's not actually your fault that you (or others you know) have found it difficult to stick with your healthier eating and regular exercise goals? If so, in what ways? If not, why not?

2. Have you ever initiated regular exercise and/or healthier eating plans when you're in a "motivation bubble"? If so, what happened?

3. Do you think you're more of a habiter or unhabiter when it comes to healthy behaviors? How might knowing this help you with your eating or exercise goals?

4. Could you relate to any of the four Decision Disruptors, or Decision TRAPs (Temptation, Rebellion, Accommodation, and Perfection), and if so, which ones challenge you the most?

5. Which ideas from *The Joy Choice* might help you prevent or successfully deal with your biggest Decision TRAPs?

6. Did the book's ideas give you any insights into how you might prevent or overcome the most challenging decision disruptors you face to making healthier choices?

7. In what ways has all-or-nothing thinking gotten in your way with exercise and healthy eating?

8. How did learning about the "choice point" concept (situations that arise that tend to derail our eating or exercise plans) impact how you confront unexpected challenges to your eating or exercise plans?

9. Picking the "perfect *imperfect* option" at an exercise or eating choice point is the recipe for sustainable success for most people. Does this idea feel like a relief and helpful, or does it feel just plain wrong, like it's going to take you in the wrong direction? Why do you feel that way?

10. Have you tried using the POP! decision tool in your life, and if so, what have you been learning?

11. Now that you have read *The Joy Choice*, what do you think is the single idea that might be most helpful to you as you move forward on your journey of lasting change with healthier eating and/or exercise?

12. After reading the book, what are some new insights about why you or others you know have had difficulty sustaining exercise and/or sticking with a more intentional way of eating?

13. *The Joy Choice* identifies four core Decision Disruptors so we could easily remember them, Temptation, Rebellion, Accommodation, and Perfection, or T.R.A.P. In addition to being easy to remember, what benefits might there be from naming our specific decision TRAPs, right in the moment of a challenging choice?

14. In what ways does having the POP decision process include the concept of "play" influence our frame of mind at choice points? How might that influence the process of making a choice?

15. Why does *The Joy Choice* suggest that changing our behavior in sustainable ways is actually *"learning"* change?

INDEX